D0891432

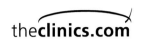

HEMATOLOGY/ ONCOLOGY CLINICS OF NORTH AMERICA

Hodgkin's Lymphoma: New Insights in an Old Disease

GUEST EDITORS
Volker Diehl, MD, Andreas Engert, MD, and Daniel Re, MD

October 2007 • Volume 21 • Number 5

SAUNDERS

An Imprint of Elsevier, Inc.
PHILADELPHIA   LONDON   TORONTO   MONTREAL   SYDNEY   TOKYO

W.B. SAUNDERS COMPANY
A Division of Elsevier Inc.

Elsevier Inc. • 1600 John F. Kennedy Boulevard • Suite 1800 • Philadelphia, Pennsylvania 19103-2899

http://www.hemonc.theclinics.com

HEMATOLOGY/ONCOLOGY CLINICS
OF NORTH AMERICA   Volume 21, Number 5
October 2007   ISSN 0889-8588
Editor: Kerry Holland   ISBN-13: 978-1-4160-5081-0
                                                ISBN-10: 1-4160-5081-7

Copyright © 2007 by Elsevier Inc. All rights reserved. No part of this publication may be reproduced or transmitted in any form or by any means, electronic or mechanical, including photocopy, recording, or any information retrieval system, without written permission from the publisher.

Single photocopies of single articles may be made for personal use as allowed by national copyright laws. Permission of the publisher and payment of a fee is required for all other photocopying, including multiple or systematic copying, copying for advertising or promotional purposes, resale, and all forms of document delivery. Special rates are available for educational institutions that wish to make photocopies for non-profit educational classroom use. Permission may be sought directly from Elsevier's Global Rights Department in Oxford, UK: phone 215-239-3804 or +44 (0)1865 843830, fax +44 (0)1865 853333, email healthpermissions@elsevier.com. Requests may also be completed online via the Elsevier homepage (http://www.elsevier.com/permissions). In the USA, users may clear permissions and make payments through the Copyright Clearance Center, Inc., 222 Rosewood Drive, Danvers, MA 01923, USA; phone: (978) 750-8400, fax: (978) 750-4744, and in the UK through the Copyright Licensing Agency Rapid Clearance Service (CLARCS), 90 Tottenham Court Road, London W1P 0LP, UK; phone: (+44) 171 436 5931; fax: (+44) 171 436 3986. Others countries may have a local reprographic rights agency for payments.

Reprints: For copies of 100 or more, of articles in this publication, please contact the Commercial Reprints Department, Elsevier Inc., 360 Park Avenue South, New York, New York 10010-1710. Tel. (212) 633-3813; Fax: (212) 462-1935; e-mail: reprints@elsevier.com.

The ideas and opinions expressed in *Hematology/Oncology Clinics of North America* do not necessarily reflect those of the Publisher. The Publisher does not assume any responsibility for any injury and/or damage to persons or property arising out of or related to any use of the material contained in this periodical. The reader is advised to check the appropriate medical literature and the product information currently provided by the manufacturer of each drug to be administered to verify the dosage, the method and duration of administration, or contraindications. It is the responsibility of the treating physician or other health care professional, relying on independent experience and knowledge of the patient, to determine drug dosages and the best treatment of the patient. Mention of any product in this issue should not be construed as endorsement by the contributors, editors, or the Publisher of the product or manufacturers' claims.

Hematology/Oncology Clinics (ISSN 0889-8588) is published bimonthly by Elsevier Inc., 360 Park Avenue South, New York, NY 10010-1710. Months of issue are February, April, June, August, October, and December. Business and Editorial Offices: 1600 John F. Kennedy Blvd., Suite 1800, Philadelphia, PA 19103-2899. Customer Service Office: 6277 Sea Harbor Drive, Orlando, FL 32887-4800. Periodicals postage paid at New York, NY and additional mailing offices. Subscription prices are $238.00 per year (US individuals), $356.00 per year (US institutions), $119.00 per year (US students), $270.00 per year (Canadian individuals), $427.00 per year (Canadian institutions), $151.00 per year (Canadian students), $302.00 per year (international individuals), $427.00 per year (international institutions), $151.00 per year (international students). International air speed delivery is included in all *Clinics* subscription prices. All prices are subject to change without notice. **POSTMASTER:** Send address changes to *Hematology/Oncology Clinics of North America*, Elsevier Periodicals Customer Service, 6277 Sea Harbor Drive, Orlando, FL 32887-4800. Customer Service: 1-800-654-2452 (US). From outside of the US, call 1-407-345-4000.

Hematology/Oncology Clinics of North America is covered in *Index Medicus, EMBASE/Excerpta Medica*, and *BIOSIS*.

Printed in the United States of America.

Hodgkin's Lymphoma: New Insights in an Old Disease

GUEST EDITORS

VOLKER DIEHL, MD, Emeritus Professor of Medicine, Department of Internal Medicine I, Haus Lebenswert, University Hospital of Cologne, Cologne, Germany

ANDREAS ENGERT, MD, Professor of Medicine, Department of Internal Medicine I, University Hospital of Cologne, Cologne, Germany

DANIEL RE, MD, Head, Laboratory for Transitional Lymphoma Research, Department of Internal Medicine I, University Hospital of Cologne, Cologne, Germany

CONTRIBUTORS

BERTHE M.P. ALEMAN, MD, Phd, Radiation Oncologist, Department of Radiotherapy, The Netherlands Cancer Institute, Amsterdam, The Netherlands

LIESELOT BREPOELS, MD, Division of Nuclear Medicine, University Hospital Gasthuisberg, Leuven, Belgium

GEORGE P. CANELLOS, MD, William Rosenberg Professor of Medicine, Harvard Medical School, Dana-Farber Cancer Institute, Boston, Massachusetts

NEIL E. CAPORASO, MD, Genetic Epidemiology Branch, Division of Cancer Epidemiology and Genetics, National Cancer Institute, Department of Health and Human Services, National Institutes of Health, Bethesda, Maryland

BRUCE D. CHESON MD, Professor of Medicine; and Head of Hematology, Georgetown University Hospital, Washington, D.C.

JOSEPH M. CONNORS, MD, Clinical Professor, University of British Columbia; Chair, Lymphoma Tumour Group, British Columbia Cancer Agency, Vancouver, British Columbia, Canada

VOLKER DIEHL, MD, Emeritus Professor of Medicine, Department of Internal Medicine I, Haus Lebenswert, University Hospital of Cologne, Cologne, Germany

GUNILLA ENBLAD, MD, PhD, Professor, Department of Oncology, Radiology and Clinical Immunology, Section of Oncology, Uppsala University Hospital, Rudbeck Laboratory C11, Uppsala, Sweden

ANDREAS ENGERT, MD, Professor of Medicine, Department of Internal Medicine I, University Hospital of Cologne, Cologne, Germany

MARIE FISCHER, PhD, Department of Oncology, Radiology and Clinical Immunology, Section of Oncology, Uppsala University Hospital, Rudbeck Laboratory C11, Uppsala; Clinical Immunology and Allergy, Department of Medicine, Karolinska Institutet, Stockholm, Sweden

INGRID GLIMELIUS, MD, Department of Oncology, Radiology and Clinical Immunology, Section of Oncology, Uppsala University Hospital, Rudbeck Laboratory C11, Uppsala, Sweden

RICHARD T. HOPPE, MD, Henry S. Kaplan-Harry Lebeson Professor of Cancer Biology; and Chair, Department of Radiation Oncology, Stanford University, Stanford, California

MICHAEL HUMMEL, PhD, Institute of Pathology, Campus Benjamin Franklin, Charité–Universitätsmedizin Berlin, Hindenburgdamm, Berlin, Germany

OLA LANDGREN, MD, PhD, Genetic Epidemiology Branch, Division of Cancer Epidemiology and Genetics, National Cancer Institute, Department of Health and Human Services, National Institutes of Health, Bethesda, Maryland

DAVID A. MACDONALD, MD, Assistant Professor, Division of Hematology, QEII Health Sciences Centre, Halifax, Nova Scotia, Canada

STEPHAN MATHAS, MD, Max-Delbrück-Center for Molecular Medicine; Hematology, Oncology and Tumor Immunology, Charité, Medical University Berlin, Campus Virchow-Klinikum, Campus Berlin-Buch, Berlin, Germany

DANIEL MOLIN, MD, PhD, Department of Oncology, Radiology and Clinical Immunology, Section of Oncology, Uppsala University Hospital, Rudbeck Laboratory C11, Uppsala, Sweden

GUNNAR NILSSON, PhD, Professor, Clinical Immunology and Allergy, Department of Medicine, Karolinska Institutet, Stockholm, Sweden

JOHN RAEMAEKERS, MD, PhD, Department of Medicine, Division of Hematology, University Hospital of Nijmegen, Nijmegen, The Netherlands

DANIEL RE, MD, Head, Laboratory for Transitional Lymphoma Research, Department of Internal Medicine I, University Hospital of Cologne, Cologne, Germany

LENA SPECHT, MD, PhD, Chief Oncologist; and Associate Professor, Departments of Oncology and Haematology, The Finsen Centre, Rigshospitalet, Copenhagen University Hospital, Copenhagen, Denmark

SIGRID STROOBANTS, MD, PhD, Professor, Division of Nuclear Medicine, University Hospital Gasthuisberg, Leuven, Belgium

CONTRIBUTORS continued

ANNA SUREDA, MD, PhD, Department of Hematology, Clinical Hematology Division, Hospital de la Santa Creu i Sant Pau, Antoni Maria i Claret, Barcelona, Spain

FLORA E. VAN LEEUWEN, PhD, Head, Department of Epidemiology, The Netherlands Cancer Institute, Amsterdam, The Netherlands

Hodgkin's Lymphoma: New Insights in an Old Disease

Hodgkin's lymphoma is a highly enigmatic lymphoma disease that still covers most of its secrets up to now. Much effort has been made to successfully wrest at least some of the pathogenetic particularities. The current diagnostic criteria are well established allowing hematopathologists to make a clear-cut distinction from other lymphomas in almost all cases. Although classic Hodgkin's lymphoma is curable in the vast majority of cases by treatment with highly aggressive drugs with or without radiotherapy, further molecular studies may lead to the identification of therapeutic targets that enable a more tailored treatment with fewer side effects.

It has been shown that differentiated lymphoid cells can display a broad developmental potential and might even differentiate into other cell types. Recent data implicate such processes in the pathogenesis of classical Hodgkin's lymphoma (HL). In the malignant, B cell–derived Hodgkin's and Reed-Sternberg (HRS) cells of HL the expression of B cell–specific genes is lost, and B lineage–inappropriate genes are upregulated. Experimental evidence has been presented in recent years that functional disruption of the B lineage–specific transcription factor program contributes to this process. HRS cells might be reprogrammed into cells resembling undifferentiated progenitor cells, which might offer an explanation for the unique HL phenotype and demonstrate a high degree of plasticity of human lymphoid cells.

The innate immune system is our first line of defense against danger signals but in Hodgkin's lymphoma the role seems opposite, favoring malignant development. In this article we describe interactions between Hodgkin's and Reed-Sternberg cells and the cells of the innate immune system: eosinophils, mast cells, neutrophils, and macrophages. These cells clearly contribute to the pathogenesis of this disease and to the prognosis. Cytokines and chemokines released from the activated immune cells probably promote tumor cell growth and survival along with angiogenesis. Mast cells and eosinophils seem also to contribute to the fibrosis that is so characteristic for nodular sclerosis.

Epstein-Barr virus (EBV) has remained the main candidate suggested as the infection causing Hodgkin's lymphoma for several years. However, EBV genome has been found only within the tumor in about 20%–40% of Hodgkin's lymphoma cases with a prior diagnosis of infectious mononucleosis. Recently, autoimmune and related conditions have drawn attention to a potential role for immune-related and inflammatory conditions in the etiology and pathogenesis of the malignancy. Evidence from multiple affected families from case series, a twin study, a case-control study, and population-based registry studies implicate a role for genetic factors. Simultaneously, data from Eastern Asia and among Chinese immigrants in North America indicate increasing incidence trends for Hodgkin's lymphoma being associated with westernization. These results emphasize an interaction between environmental and genetic risk factors in Hodgkin's lymphoma.

Clinical trials are critical to the development of newer and more effective treatments. Standardized response criteria are essential to assess and compare the activity of various therapies within and among studies and to facilitate the evaluation of new treatments by regulatory agencies. The International Harmonization Project developed revised guidelines with the goal of improved comparability among studies, leading to accelerated new agent development resulting in the rapid availability of improved therapies for patients who have lymphoma. Modifications of these recommendations are expected as new information and improved technologies become available.

Is [¹⁸F]fluorodeoxyglucose Positron Emission Tomography the Ultimate Tool for Response and Prognosis Assessment?

Lieselot Brepoels and Sigrid Stroobants

[¹⁸F]fluorodeoxyglucose positron emission tomography (FDG-PET) is currently the most accurate and reliable tool for the assessment of response in Hodgkin's lymphoma (HL). FDG-PET is superior to conventional imaging techniques for detection of residual disease at the end of treatment, especially in the presence of a residual mass, a frequent finding in HL. FDG-PET response assessment has also a high predictive value early after the initiation of therapy. However, whether risk-adapted treatment strategies based on FDG-PET may also improve patient outcome remains to be proved.

New Strategies for the Treatment of Early Stages of Hodgkin's Lymphoma

David A. Macdonald and Joseph M. Connors

The treatment of early or limited-stage Hodgkin's lymphoma continues to evolve. With the likelihood of cure of the lymphoma approaching 95% it has become increasingly necessary to balance improved effectiveness of treatment with minimization of troublesome late toxicity. Carefully crafted treatment strategies based on optimal combinations of brief chemotherapy and involved-field radiation or even reliance on brief chemotherapy alone for carefully selected patients have emerged as the most attractive approaches to achieve this important balance.

Do We Need an Early Unfavorable (Intermediate) Stage of Hodgkin's Lymphoma?

Lena Specht and John Raemaekers

The outcome of patients who have early unfavorable or intermediate-stage Hodgkin's lymphoma has greatly improved. The increasing efficacy of chemotherapy and late toxic effects of wide-field radiotherapy justify the careful testing of the new involved-node radiotherapy principle in the combined-modality approach. For the purpose of tailoring treatment to the individual patient we need more accurate measures, preferably predictive factors that may tell us how the individual patient should be treated. The result of an early positron emission tomography scan with fluorodeoxyglucose may well become the major new treatment-related guidance for an individually tailored treatment approach.

New Strategies for the Treatment of Advanced-Stage Hodgkin's Lymphoma

Volker Diehl, Andreas Engert, and Daniel Re

In 2007, patients who have Hodgkin's lymphoma, even in advanced stages, have a better than 85% chance of being cured of their disease if adequate therapy is given at the outset. Most ongoing or planned international studies tailor therapy according to the needs of the individual patient, also accounting for anatomic stage, tumor burden, age, gender, and biologic host factors that affect prognosis. With this approach it might be possible to use less aggressive treatment regimens for the lower-risk groups and limit the use of the more aggressive dose- and time-intensified/dense regimens for the higher-risk groups. With this individualized approach it might be possible to yield higher cure rates and simultaneously reduce the risk for late complications and mortality.

A history of the treatment of Hodgkin's disease with radiation therapy and chemotherapy is presented. Studies are reviewed examining treatment for favorable and unfavorable presentation of stage I–II disease, stage III–IV disease, and relapsed disease. In this era of combined-modality therapy we have reached the point of near-total conquest of Hodgkin's lymphoma, but challenges remain. Directions for future research are discussed.

Relapse or progression following therapy for Hodgkin's lymphoma occurs in 10% to 60% of patients depending on initial clinical stage. Patterns of failure in advanced disease determine prognosis of salvage therapy. Progression or early relapse after less than 12 months requires intensive salvage therapy. Only late, isolated, asymptomatic relapse, which occurs in less than 25% of those relapsing from systemic therapy, can be treated with conventional-dose chemotherapy with or without radiation. Overall about 40% to 50% of relapses from advanced disease can be salvaged with higher percentages for patients relapsing from early stage disease.

Newly diagnosed patients who have advanced-stage Hodgkin's lymphoma have an excellent prognosis because most of them can be cured with initial treatment. In contrast, the prognosis for patients relapsing after first-line therapy with either combination chemotherapy or chemotherapy followed by radiotherapy remains poor in many cases. In most of these cases, high-dose chemotherapy and autologous stem cell trans-plantation (ASCT) is currently considered to be the treatment of choice. However, results of ASCT in primary refractory patients are poor and new therapeutic alternatives should be sought for these patients. Allogeneic stem cell transplantation has been used increasingly in relapsed or refractory Hodgkin's lymphoma patients, with the introduction of re-duced-intensity conditioning protocols.

The cure rate of patients who have Hodgkin's lymphoma (HL) amounts to 80% or more because of risk-adapted treatment using modern chemotherapy and radiotherapy schedules. In this article we describe important late effects after treatment of HL and how we expect the long-term burden of patients who have HL to change applying modern treatments. Because treatment always has side effects to some extent, awareness of possible late effects after treatment remains important for patients and treating physicians.

HEMATOLOGY/ONCOLOGY CLINICS
OF NORTH AMERICA

ELSEVIER
SAUNDERS

THE CLINICS ARE NOW AVAILABLE ONLINE!

Access your subscription at:
http://www.theclinics.com

Preface

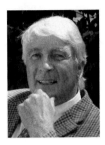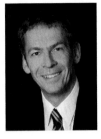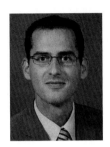

Volker Diehl, MD
Andreas Engert, MD
Daniel Re, MD
Guest Editors

H odgkin's Lymphoma (HL) is one of the best curable cancers in adulthood. Today, patients in different stages can be cured with modern
risk-, and response-adapted treatment strategies in 85%–95 % of cases.
Over the past 60 years, however, the risk of failure changed for the patient to
survive the diagnosis of HL. Before 1960, the high risk of dying from the
tumor threatened the patient. Later on, invasive diagnostic procedures such
as exploratory laparotomy and splenectomy put patients at risk because they
caused high rates of moribidity and sometimes mortality. With the advent of
large field radiotherapy in the 1970s, higher survival rates were achieved at
the cost of short-term and long-term, potentially fatal, sequelae. This risk of late
effects secondary to aggressive treatment is increased further with combined
modality approaches applied from the 1980s to present. Currently, one of
the highest risks for HL patients is not getting the best risk-adapted therapy
from the very beginning of diagnosis.

This issue of *Hematology/Oncology Clinics of North America* gives an overview on
current therapeutic and diagnostic strategies supporting the doctor in private
practices and in the academic institution to diagnose and treat HL patients
according to their personal needs and individual risk profiles using the most
effective and least toxic strategy. Further, the overviews presented in this issue
address the pathology, biology, molecular-pathogenesis, and epidemiology
of HL. Novel diagnostic tools and new therapeutic strategies developed to
maintain high cure rates and reduce long-term toxicities in cancer survivors
also are discussed.

0889-8588/07/$ – see front matter
doi:10.1016/j.hoc.2007.07.006 © 2007 Elsevier Inc. All rights reserved.
hemonc.theclinics.com

The advent of fluorodeoxyglucose-positron emission tomography as a re-sponse- and a prognosis-predicting tool at an early point in the carrier of an HL patient, enables clinicians to tailor therapy according to the individual risk of failure to induction therapy and prevent overtreatment and/or undertreatment.

The unresolved question whether or not we need an intermediate (early unfavorable) stage allocation in HL is addressed in detail. The role of adjuvant or consolidative radiation in conjunction with chemotherapy is discussed, and it is questioned whether the doctor will become the most prominent risk factor for HL patients in the future if he/she is not familiar with the most efficacious therapeutic tools, and even more if he/she is not willing to put a patient in the best available clinical trial.

As of 2007, each HL patient has the right to be cured in the most suitable time with the best strategy available if he/she has access to modern cancer care. We hope you find that this issue provides the information and tools to accomplish this goal.

Volker Diehl, MD
Department of Internal Medicine I
Haus Lebenswert
University Hospital of Cologne
Kerpenerstr. 62
50931 Cologne, Germany

Andreas Engert, MD
Daniel Re, MD
Department of Internal Medicine I
University Hospital of Cologne
Kerpenerstr. 62
50931 Cologne, Germany

E-mail addresses: v.diehl@uni-koeln.de, a.engert@uni-koeln.de,
daniel.re@uni-koeln.de

World Health Organization and Beyond: New Aspects in the Pathology of an Old Disease

Michael Hummel, PhD

Institute of Pathology, Campus Benjamin Franklin, Charité–Universitätsmedizin Berlin,
Hindenburgdamm 30, D-12200 Berlin, Germany

HISTORICAL CONSIDERATIONS

The history of Hodgkin's lymphoma is one of the most fascinating stories in medicine beginning before the first concise description by Thomas Hodgkin [1] in 1832. Before his publication, several "practical morbid anatomists" mentioned single cases with an appearance similar to the cases recognized by Hodgkin as an independent disease entity. Without knowledge of the description by Hodgkin, Wilks [2] published in the year 1856 15 cases (including 1 or 2 cases described by Hodgkin) with the same features as the cases previously identified by Hodgkin. Wilks was not aware of the previous work of Hodgkin when he documented his observations, however. Because he suggested that this disease entity deserved a distinct name, the idea to call it "Wilks disease" was obvious. When Wilks became aware that he was not the first to recognize these cases with a particular anatomy he added a comment to his already completed paper. In this comment he expressed his regret that he overlooked Hodgkin's observation. One major reason for his ignorance was that Hodgkin failed to affix a distinct name to this disease entity. Wilks [3] was generous enough to honor the discovery by Hodgkin in his publication of 1865, however, with the suggestion to use the term "Hodgkin's disease" henceforth. In parallel and in addition to the discussions and publications of Wilks and Hodgkin, several further apparently independent descriptions of single cases supported the value of subsuming these characteristic lymph node swellings as one single and distinct entity [4,5].

Because the above recapitulated discoveries were made by macroscopic observations alone, a controversial discussion broke out when other malignancies were described demonstrating similar anatomic features as those described by Wilks and Hodgkin. In 1872 and 1878 Langhans [6] and Greenfield [7], respectively, defined the histologic characteristics of Hodgkin's disease for the first time. They both highlighted the peculiar presence of multinucleated giant cells

E-mail address: michael.hummel@charite.de

0889-8588/07/$ – see front matter
doi:10.1016/j.hoc.2007.06.015
© 2007 Elsevier Inc. All rights reserved.
hemonc.theclinics.com

harboring up to 12 nuclei. Despite this first description of the cells characteristic for Hodgkin's disease by Langhans and Greenfield, Sternberg [8] and Reed [9] are generally credited with the first description, most likely because of their more comprehensive depiction supported by detailed drawings.

The particular histologic features in combination with the anatomic characteristics convincingly justified delineating Hodgkin's disease from other types of lymph node swellings. A precise reevaluation of the cases published by Hodgkin and Wilks disclosed that not all of the cases still available displayed the characteristic histology [10] and it became apparent that the macroscopic consideration alone was not sufficient for the reliable diagnosis of Hodgkin's disease. The histologic unconfirmed historical cases were mainly tuberculosis, systemic lymphocytosis, or syphilis, which may mimic from an anatomic point of view a true Hodgkin's disease.

After this initial discovery and basic definition of Hodgkin's disease, a period of several decades followed in which many more cases were collected leading to a consolidation and an extension of knowledge. In 1947 Jackson and Parker [11] made a first attempt to classify the different types of Hodgkin's disease. Mainly three groups have been identified in this classification: Hodgkin's granuloma (main group), Hodgkin's sarcoma (great abundance of pleomorphic and anaplastic Reed-Sternberg cells) and Hodgkin's paragranuloma (small number of atypical cells and slow clinical course).

The classification of Parker and Jackson was preferentially in use until Lukes and Butler [12] suggested a largely modified categorization of the cases of Hodgkin's disease, which was presented 1966 at the Rye conference, New York. This classification distinguished four different types of Hodgkin's disease: lymphocyte predominant, mixed cellularity, nodular sclerosis, and lymphocyte depleted.

The Rye Classification was commonly applied until the introduction of the Revised European-American Lymphoma (R.E.A.L.) Classification, which divided Hodgkin's disease into main categories, namely classic Hodgkin's disease and lymphocyte-predominant Hodgkin's disease [13]. This distinction was obvious because lymphocyte-predominant Hodgkin's disease differs consistently from classic Hodgkin's disease in immunophenotype, morphology, and clinical behavior. Within the classic type of Hodgkin's disease a further subdivision was suggested by the R.E.A.L. classification that was based on the histologic differences already recognized by Lukes and Bulter [12]: mixed cellularity, nodular sclerosis, and lymphocyte depleted. In addition to these subtypes of classic Hodgkin's disease, lymphocyte-rich classic Hodgkin's disease was introduced as a new and provisional disease entity. In previous classifications this new entity had been lumped together with lymphocyte-predominant Hodgkin's disease because of similar histologic features. Careful immunophenotypic considerations and clinical features justified its separation as a distinct subtype of classic Hodgkin's disease.

The currently effective classification of Hodgkin's disease was established by the World Health Organization (WHO) Classification of Hematopoietic and

Lymphoid Neoplasms (2001) (Box 1) [14]. The WHO classification accepted the subdivision into two major Hodgkin's lymphoma categories as established by the R.E.A.L. classification. In addition, the term Hodgkin's disease was replaced by the term Hodgkin's lymphoma. Finally, the provisional lymphocyte-rich classic Hodgkin's disease category of the R.E.A.L. classification was formally accepted as a distinct subgroup in WHO classification termed classic lymphocyte-rich Hodgkin's lymphoma.

HISTOLOGIC SUBTYPING OF CLASSIC HODGKIN'S LYMPHOMA

As evident from the different subtypes of classic Hodgkin's lymphoma there is no concordant pattern of lymph node involvement. Furthermore, the extent of effacement of the physiologic lymph node architecture can range from a partial involvement consisting of only a few atypical cells to a total involvement with a complete effacement of normal lymph node architecture. A consistent characteristic that is indispensable for diagnosis of classic Hodgkin's lymphoma is the presence of the disease-defining Hodgkin and Reed-Sternberg (HRS) cells. These cells might occur as the mononuclear variant (Hodgkin's cells) or as the multinuclear variant (Reed-Sternberg cells). Usually a mixture of the mononuclear Hodgkin's cells and the multinuclear Hodgkin's and Reed-Sternberg cells coexist within the neoplastic lesions. The mere presence of HRS cells is not sufficient for the diagnosis of a classic Hodgkin's lymphoma, however; diagnosis requires in addition a histologic growth pattern typical of Hodgkin's lymphoma.

The histologic growth patterns are inhomogeneously distributed among the cases of Hodgkin's lymphoma. The most common type is the nodular sclerosis subtype, which is found in developed countries in approximately 50% to 60% of cases. Mixed cellularity subtype composes approximately 30%, whereas lymphocyte-rich classic Hodgkin's lymphoma represents only 4% to 5% of the cases and lymphocyte-depleted is rare, occurring in less than 1% of the cases. In a fraction of the 5% to 10% of the classic Hodgkin's lymphoma cases a reliable subclassification is not possible because of overlapping features or scarcity of the diagnostic material (ie, fine needle biopsies).

Box 1: World Health Organization classification of Hodgkin's lymphoma

Nodular lymphocyte-predominant Hodgkin's lymphoma

Classic Hodgkin's lymphoma

    Nodular sclerosis

    Mixed cellularity

    Lymphocyte-rich

    Lymphocyte-depleted

Nodular Sclerosis Subtype of Classic Hodgkin's Lymphoma

The most prominent feature of the nodular sclerosis (NS) subtype of classic Hodgkin's lymphoma is the presence of collagenous bands that enclose nodules of lymphoid cells with variable numbers of HRS cells embedded in a reactive infiltrate [12–14]. The HRS cells that are recognized as lacunar cells in a substantial number of cases might be present as cell sheets [15]. These lacunar cells show large, multilobated or irregular nuclei with small nucleoli, pale cytoplasm, and finely dispersed chromatin. The reactive infiltrate is composed of numerous eosinophils and neutrophils in addition to lymphocytes, whereas histiocytes and plasma cells are less prevalent. Sometimes fibrohistiocytic foci are found that may even largely replace the tissue. Notably, para-apoptotic HRS cells (mummified HRS cells) are nearly exclusively found in the NS subtype of classic Hodgkin's lymphoma [16]. A previously suggested grading system for the subdivision of the NS subtype of classic Hodgkin's lymphoma (NS1 and NS2) based on (1) the pleomorphic or reticular lymphocyte depletion, and/or (2) the fibrohistiocytic lymphocyte depletion, and/or (3) the presence of highly anaplastic and bizarre HRS cells was abolished because no different clinical outcome was observed between NS1 and NS2 [17,18].

Mixed Cellularity Subtype of Classic Hodgkin's Lymphoma

In Western countries the mixed cellularity (MC) subtype represents the second most common category of classic Hodgkin's lymphoma (~30%), whereas in developing countries around 50% of the classic Hodgkin's lymphoma cases present as MC subtype. A characteristic feature of this subtype is the heterogeneous mixture of small lymphocytes, eosinophils, neutrophils, (epithelioid and nonepithelioid) histiocytes, and plasma cells in which a variable number of HRS cells are embedded [12–14]. The histologic pattern of the MC subtype is broad, ranging from diffuse to suggestively nodular but without the band-forming sclerosis. Because MC subtype cases may display overlapping features with other classic Hodgkin's lymphoma subtypes, a clear delineation, especially from lymphocyte-rich and lymphocyte-depleted subtypes, is difficult or impossible in some instances.

Lymphocyte-Rich Subtype of Classic Hodgkin's Lymphoma

The R.E.A.L. classification was the first to suggest distinguishing between lymphocyte-predominant Hodgkin's lymphoma and classic Hodgkin's lymphoma of the lymphocyte-rich (LR) subtype [12–14]. Most LR classic lymphoma cases present with a nodular background in which a variable number of HRS cells, sometime with popcorn morphology, are admixed together with numerous histiocytes. Usually eosinophils and neutrophils are largely missing [19].

Lymphocyte-Depleted Subtype of Classic Hodgkin's Lymphoma

Initially described by Lukes and Butler [12] and confirmed by the Rye conference, the lymphocyte-depleted (LD) subtype of classic Hodgkin's lymphoma represents by far the most rare variant (less than 1% of all cases). The lymphoid component is underrepresented, whereas a large number of HRS cells are present. In the reticular variant of LD classic Hodgkin's lymphoma the HRS cells are abundant with a bizarre morphology, whereas the diffuse fibrosis variant is characterized by an extensive unorganized fibrosis that seems to envelop the individual HRS cells [20].

NODULAR LYMPHOCYTE-PREDOMINANT HODGKIN'S LYMPHOMA

Until the introduction of the R.E.A.L. classification the nodular lymphocyte-predominant (LP) Hodgkin's lymphomas have been merged together with the lymphocyte-rich (LR) classic Hodgkin's lymphoma [13]. This delineation from classic type of Hodgkin's lymphoma is justified not only on histologic or immunophenotypic grounds but also from a clinical point of view because LP Hodgkin's lymphoma, which accounts for approximately 7% of all Hodgkin's lymphomas in Western countries, is characterized by an indolent clinical course.

The atypical cells of LP Hodgkin's lymphoma (termed popcorn cells or L&H cells) differ from HRS cells in that they share similarities with centroblasts with small nucleoli, often in the vicinity of the nuclear membrane, and with polylobulated nuclei. The growth pattern of LP Hodgkin's lymphoma is usually nodular with sometimes diffuse areas; a predominant diffuse growth pattern is rare. The reactive background consists of mainly lymphocytes with a variable number of histiocytes and rare plasma cells. Eosinophils and neutrophils are infrequently present in LP Hodgkin's lymphoma and occasional sclerosis may mimic a classic Hodgkin's lymphoma of NS subtype in some cases [21].

Immuonphenotypically the L&H cells of LP Hodgkin's lymphoma are consistently strongly positive for CD20 and other B-cell characteristic markers and often display an overexpression of OCT2 that is even stronger than the expression in reactive B cells [22]. Consequently, L&H cells show a strong immunoglobulin (Ig) heavy chain gene expression in most instances. Single-cell analysis of L&H cells revealed functional Ig rearrangement which, in common with classic Hodgkin's lymphoma, carries high loads of somatic Ig hypermutations [23–25]. Because of the indolent clinical course, which includes spontaneous regression without treatment in many cases, a polyclonal origin of the L&H cells was often suggested. Again single-cell analysis was able to unequivocally demonstrate that L&H cells are clonal and as a consequence of their germinal center origin carry ongoing somatic Ig hypermutations.

CD30, a hallmark of classic Hodgkin's lymphoma [26], is absent from the L&H cells of LP Hodgkin's lymphoma with rare exceptions [21]. In addition, the J-chain is expressed in the vast majority of LP Hodgkin's lymphoma cases but not in classic Hodgkin's lymphoma, with rare exceptions. Additional characteristics to distinguish LP Hodgkin's lymphoma from classic Hodgkin's lymphoma are LMP1 and CD15 [27], which are both found in a significant proportion of classic Hodgkin's lymphoma but are not described to by expressed by L&H cells [14].

HODGKIN'S AND REED-STERNBERG CELLS: THE TUMOR CELLS OF CLASSIC HODGKIN'S LYMPHOMA

The cellular origin of the HRS cells of classic Hodgkin's lymphoma was for a long time a mystery. Two major reasons account for this exceptional situation: (1) the scarcity of the HRS cells in affected tissues, and (2) the absence of a consistent marker profile. Because the HRS cells are usually underrepresented in most cases, detailed molecular analyses are not possible based on whole tissue extracts. This difficult situation raised much speculation around the cellular counterpart of the HRS cells, ranging from macrophages [28], myeloid cells [29], follicular dendritic cells [30], and interdigitating cells [31], to activated B or T cells.

The hope that the use of monoclonal antibodies would clarify the cellular nature of the HRS cells was in vain. No consistent pattern was initially found; instead overlapping and/or contradictory antigenic features were observed in most cases. The first consistent feature present in virtually all cases was the expression of CD30, a member of the tumor necrosis factor receptor family [32,33]. The expression of CD30 provided clear evidence that the HRS cells derive from lymphoid cells [34]. It was unclear, however, whether B or T cells may represent the cellular counterpart of the HRS cells because CD30 can be expressed by activated B cells and activated T cells.

The conclusion that the expression of CD30 identifies lymphoid cells as the counterpart of HRS cells was not generally accepted because most classic Hodgkin's lymphoma cases do not display markers typical of B or T cells. The sometimes impassioned discussion around the cellular nature of the HRS cells continued.

The introduction of the polymerase chain reaction (PCR) and its application to the analysis of rearranged Ig and T-cell receptor (TCR) genes offered the opportunity to unequivocally confirm or exclude the lymphoid nature of the HRS cells. Initial attempts using DNA from whole tissue extracts demonstrated clonally rearranged IgH genes in approximately one third of the classic Hodgkin's lymphoma cases investigated, leaving much room for ongoing speculation [35].

Only when techniques became available to isolate single HRS cells from tissue sections and to analyze the antigen receptor rearrangement configuration by PCR could their cellular derivation could be undoubtedly clarified: Almost all cases of classic Hodgkin's lymphoma derive from B cells that were clonally related [36–39]. Classic Hodgkin's lymphoma cases that derive from T cells are extremely rare, accounting for less than 2% of all cases [40,41].

Detailed analysis of the rearranged Ig genes amplified from the HRS cells demonstrated that they usually carried high loads of somatic Ig mutations [39,42]. This fact identified the HRS cells as derivatives of germinal center or postgerminal center B cells. Although the B-cell nature of the HRS cells was now broadly accepted there was again an emotional discussion regarding the reasons for the absence of Ig RNA and protein expression and for the absence of other B cell–typical antigens. Based on the presence of the so-called "crippling" mutations in the rearranged Ig genes of approximately 25% to 30% of the classic Hodgkin's lymphoma cases, it was suggested that these alterations might prevent the expression of functional Ig genes. This suggestion ignores that the vast majority of classic Hodgkin's lymphomas carry intact Ig rearrangements and that not only do HRS cells lack Ig but in addition they lack an expression of most other B-cell antigens in nearly all instances [39]. Once again, there is much room for further worldwide discussion.

The Discrepant Phenotypic and Genotypic Face of the Hodgkin's and Reed-Sternberg Cells

In the search for an alternative explanation for the absence of a B-cell phenotype of the HRS cells, B-cell characteristic transcription factors attracted much attention. Most discussion focused around the B-cell transcription factor OCT2 and its cofactor BOB.1 [22]. As demonstrated by immunohistology, OCT2 and BOB.1 are absent from the vast majority of classic Hodgkin's lymphomas or were mutually expressed in the remaining cases. Reintroduction of OCT2 and/or BOB.1 in Hodgkin's-derived cell lines demonstrated that exogenous Ig promoters can be reactivated by this approach but a reactivation of the endogenous Ig genes or other B-cell antigens could not be achieved [43]. One reason for this inability to reactivate the expression of the Ig genes by overexpression of OCT2 and BOB.1 in Hodgkin's-derived cell lines might be inaccessibility of transcription factor binding sites because of closed heterochromatin at the promoter of the Ig genes [44]. In addition, hypermethylation of the Ig gene promoters and other B-cell characteristic genes might contribute to the particular immunophenotype of the HRS cells.

This epigenetic idea fits nicely with the notion that the event leading to the Hodgkin's phenotype is a single event that occurs in a short time frame [45]. The treatment of Hodgkin's-derived cell lines with demethylating agents led to only minor effects on the reactivation of the Ig expression or other B-cell characteristic antigens. As demonstrated by the author's unpublished experiments, a reactivation above background cannot be evoked by this treatment when the expression levels were analyzed by quantitative real-time PCR.

Recently we demonstrated that aberrant expression of B-cell–inappropriate transcription factors, such as ID2 and ABF1, expressed in primary HRS cells and in Hodgkin's-derived cell lines [46]. Because these transcription factors are known to repress the B-cell expression program in early lymphoid development, a reprogramming of the transformed HRS cells toward B cell precursor cells became conceivable. This idea is supported by our observation that overexpression of ABF1 or ID2 in B-cell lines is able to at least partially repress the B-cell expression program in these cells.

The Exceptional Immunophenotype of the Hodgkin's and Reed-Sternberg Cells

Gene expression profiling of Hodgkin's-derived cell lines revealed a heterogeneous picture with a down-regulation of almost all B-cell– and T-cell–related genes. In addition, detailed inspection of the profiles provided evidence that there is an enormous heterogeneity among the Hodgkin's cell lines analyzed. When compared with the in vivo situation similar findings became apparent. B-cell characteristic markers, such as CD19, CD20, CD22, and CD79a, are expressed only in a fraction (20%–25%) of classic Hodgkin's lymphoma cases [47]. Moreover, many of the positive cases display a weak expression that is not detectable in all HRS cells [41]. The only B-cell marker that is found in almost all classic Hodgkin's lymphoma cases is the transcription factor PAX5 [48,49]. Usually the PAX5 expression level is significantly lower in the HRS cells when compared with the surrounding reactive B cells. Despite the B-cell genotype, an expression of T-cell markers (CD2, CD3, CD4, CD5, CD8, granzyme B, TIA-1) can be observed by the HRS cells in a small proportion of cases in various combinations [50–53]. Other lineage-inappropriate makers, such as CD15 [54], Fascin [55], and Vimentin [56], are found in most cases. The transcription factor MUM1/IRF4 is strongly positive in virtually all classic Hodgkin's lymphoma cases in all HRS cells [57]. Because MUM1/IRF4 is required to shift germinal center B cells toward plasma cells [58], it is tempting to speculate that premalignant HRS cell precursors are in a (pre-) plasmacellular differentiation stage when they are hit by the transforming event. The loss of the B-cell expression program of the HRS cells is in harmony with this assumption because almost all B-cell characteristic genes are silenced in plasma cells.

The Role of Nuclear Factor κB in HRS Cells

A further consistent feature of the HRS cells is, in addition to the constant CD30 expression, the constitutive activity of the nuclear factor κB (NFκB) system [59]. NFκB is a pleiotropic transcription factor family that mediates the expression of numerous genes involved in many different functions, such as inflammation, immune response, apoptosis, and cell proliferation [60,61]. The finding of constitutive NFκB activation in HRS cells, which was initially described for Hodgkin's-derived cell lines [62], would also explain the cellular composition present in classic Hodgkin's lymphoma tissues and the expression profile of the HRS cells itself. In search for reasons for the aberrant NFκB activity in HRS cells, the NFκB inhibitors raised much interest because they were found to be defective in most Hodgkin's-derived cell lines. The assignment of this finding to primary HRS cells revealed disappointing results because of the absence of inactivation mutations in the IκB genes of the vast majority of classic Hodgkin's lymphoma cases [63–65]. To further explain the constitutive NFκB activity of the HRS cells, other defects within the NFκB system have been suggested along with a permanent activation of the NFκB system by signaling of members of the TNFR family, including CD30 and CD40 [66,67]. Currently the precise mechanism for NFκB activation in classic Hodgkin's lymphoma is still unclear. According to inhibition experiments, however, NFκB seems to play an important role in the survival of the HRS cells. Blockage of NFκB in HRS cells by a dominant negative inhibitor resulted in the down-regulation of many NFκB target genes and induction of apoptosis [68]. This finding is in line with the recent observation that the

NFκB subunit, c-REL, is also demonstrable in the nuclei of the HRS cells of most classic Hodgkin's lymphoma, indicating that NFκB is also in vivo a decisive factor for the survival of the HRS cells [69]. In addition to the consistent expression of NFκB by the HRS cell, activated caspase-3 is also found in most of the cases [69]. This finding indicates that HRS cells are permanently under the influence of apoptotic (caspase-3) and antiapoptotic (NFκB) signals, leading to a tightly balanced situation. The shift of the balance toward caspase-3 might explain the good clinical response to aggressive treatment [70].

This concurrent situation is described not only for antiapoptotic and proapoptotic molecules but also for molecules related to tumor suppressor pathways and cell cycle checkpoints. In most classic Hodgkin's lymphoma cases a constant overexpression of Hdm-2 is observed, which may lead to p53 inactivation [71]. This mechanism is able to explain the unusually low frequency of p53 mutations in classic Hodgkin's lymphoma and the p53 overexpression, but with defective p53 function. Furthermore, an overexpression of cyclin E and CDK2 is found in most classic Hodgkin's lymphoma cases. The activity of cyclin E/CDK2 complex to drive cell cycle progression into S phase is negatively regulated by p27Kip1 which, strikingly, is absent or weakly expressed in most HRS cells [72]. The overexpression of cyclin E might moreover contribute to chromosomal instability and polyploidy, hallmarks of the cells.

GENETIC ABERRATIONS

The presence of chromosomal losses and gains by comparative genomic hybridization (CGH) and genetic translocations by fluorescence in situ hybridization (FISH) are difficult to assess in classic Hodgkin's lymphoma because of the scarcity of the HRS cells. The analysis of Hodgkin's-derived cell lines by means of CGH identified many copy number changes in the cell line cells, which showed to some extent intraclonal variations [73]. There are also recurrent copy numbers on chromosome 2p and 3p involving REL and JAK2, respectively [74]. Furthermore, increased copy numbers have also been found for chromosomal regions covering cyclin D2 and MYC. Ongoing studies for the investigation of primary HRS cells are currently performed (Michael Hummel, PhD, unpublished data) to determine the presence and frequency of copy number aberrations in primary tumor cells. Most recently a comprehensive FISH study involving 230 classic Hodgkin's lymphomas found recurrent IgH rearrangement in 17% of the cases. The identifiable IgH fusion partners in the cases were c-REL, BCL6, MYC, and BCL3 [75]. In most cases the IgH fusion partners have not yet been described.

EPSTEIN-BARR VIRUS

The history of Hodgkin's disease was always accompanied by the question of whether an infectious agent plays a causal role in the pathogenesis of this disease. Many different candidates have been considered and many efforts have been undertaken to identify such an infectious agent. Most attempts revealed disappointing results, however. With the detection of the Epstein-Barr virus (EBV) a new candidate was discovered and the identification of EBV as the cause of infectious mononucleosis supported this view. Early investigations with DNA extracts from Hodgkin's tissues revealed an EBV positivity only in the minority of cases [76]. When highly sensitive PCR technology became available, the positivity rate increased to up to 80% [77,78] and more of the classic Hodgkin's lymphoma cases. Because an EBV infection was also detectable in approximately 25% of lymphoid tissues from healthy donors [77], the high detection rate in Hodgkin's lymphoma cases might represent an overestimation. This assumption was confirmed when in situ hybridizations for the detection of small noncoding EBV RNA molecules (EBER1 and EBER2) (located in the nuclei of EBV-infected cells in high copy numbers) were performed. An EBV infection of the HRS cells was present in 40% of the classic Hodgkin's lymphoma cases, whereas in the remaining cases found to be positive by EBV-PCR only an infection of a variable number of bystander cells could be observed [79,80]. Strikingly, in cases with an EBV infection of the HRS cells an infection of virtually all HRS cells could be observed without exception and this infection proved to be clonal [81]. This observation is in contrast to findings in EBV-positive non-Hodgkin's lymphomas in which the frequency is low (3%–5%) and most cases display an EBV infection in only a proportion of the tumor cells [82]. In addition to the presence of EBER, an expression of the EBV-encoded latent membrane protein 1 (LMP1) was found in the vast majority of cases, identifying this infection pattern as type 2 [83]. The EBV infection rate of classic Hodgkin's lymphoma cases from developing countries is much higher, reaching almost 100%. Notably, lymphocyte-predominant Hodgkin's lymphoma is consistently devoid of EBV infection.

The discussion about the pathogenic role of EBV continued despite only partial positivity of classic Hodgkin's lymphoma. An interesting observation supported the importance of EBV for the survival of the HRS cells at least in an early phase of the tumor cell development. Classic Hodgkin's lymphoma cases that carry crippling mutations in their clonally rearranged IgH genes are predominantly those that are EBV infected [84]. In conjunction with the observation that EBV is able to rescue nonmalignant germinal center B cells with crippling Ig mutation from cell death it is tempting to speculate that this might also be a mechanism active in an early phase of the development of classic Hodgkin's lymphoma. It remains to be elucidated which mechanisms might be involved in the pathogenesis of the EBV-negative classic Hodgkin's lymphomas.

THE ROLE OF RECEPTOR TYROSINE KINASES

Recently it was shown that several receptor protein tyrosine kinases (RTK) (PDGFRA, DDR2, RON, EPHB1, TRKA, TRKB) are expressed in a substantial number of classic Hodgkin's lymphoma cases [85]. These molecules are known as important intracellular signal transduction pathways and are closely linked to cell proliferation; it is assumed that they play an important role in the pathogenesis of many malignancies. Usually only one type of RTK is expressed in a certain tumor, which was explained by their overlapping functions. In classic Hodgkin's lymphoma cases, however, the simultaneous expression of three or more different RTKs is frequently observed. Strikingly, this RTK overexpression is predominantly found in EBV-negative classic Hodgkin's lymphoma cases [86]. It was therefore suggested that the overexpression of RTK may act in a similar way as EBV (LMP-1) in the EBV-positive cases. If the RTKs are important not only in pathogenesis of classic Hodgkin's lymphoma but also for survival of the HRS cells, an RTK-targeted therapeutic approach seems to be a promising new strategy for successful treatment of classic Hodgkin's lymphoma.

DIFFERENTIAL DIAGNOSIS

Because the diagnostic criteria, including those for classic Hodgkin's lymphoma immunophenotyping, are well established, the rate of misdiagnosis seems to be limited. There are some borderline situations that might cause misinterpretation, however. In some cases of MC classic Hodgkin's lymphoma a resemblance to infectious mononucleosis may cause diagnostic difficulties [87]. In addition, lymph node tuberculosis may be confused with classic Hodgkin's lymphoma.

Classic Hodgkin's lymphoma may be mistaken for several types of non-Hodgkin's lymphomas. Between anaplastic large cell lymphoma (ALCL) and syncytial-type NS classic Hodgkin's lymphoma, a clear-cut borderline is hard or impossible to draw, especially in Hodgkin's lymphoma cases without expression of PAX5 [88]. Another T-cell lymphoma subtype that may cause differential diagnostic problems is the occasional case of peripheral T-cell lymphoma, unspecified, which may contain CD30-positive binucleated giant cells [89].

Although the histologic features are similar between LR classic Hodgkin's lymphoma, T cell–rich B-cell lymphoma, and lymphocyte-predominant Hodgkin's lymphoma, careful reconsideration and application of selected immunophenotypic markers should be able to clarify the diagnostic difficulties in most instances [88]. The overlapping histologic and immunophenotypic features are further underscored by molecular biologic findings that demonstrate overlapping genetic features and joint characteristics in their gene expression profiles [90].

COEXISTENT B-CELL NON-HODGKIN'S LYMPHOMA

In 3% to 4% of the classic Hodgkin's lymphoma cases a simultaneous or subsequent occurrence of a non-Hodgkin's lymphoma can be observed. The coexisting non-Hodgkin's lymphomas (which range from chronic lymphocytic leukemia of B-cell type to diffuse usually large B-cell lymphoma) share no morphologic or immunophenotypic similarities with the classic Hodgkin's lymphoma in the same patient, thus fulfilling the criteria of composite lymphoma [45,91,92]. It came as surprise, however, that most of the composite lymphoma in Hodgkin's patients displayed the same IgH rearrangement. Two possibilities exist to explain these findings: (1) the Hodgkin's and the non-Hodgkin's lymphoma derive independently from the same tumor precursor cell, or (2) the Hodgkin's lymphoma developed from the non-Hodgkin's lymphoma or vice versa. Detailed single-cell analysis provided evidence in favor of the first hypothesis. As observed in a patient who had a classic Hodgkin's lymphoma and subsequent follicular lymphoma, both malignancies shared a proportion of the somatic mutations in their rearranged IgH genes and developed additional tumor-specific somatic mutations in the course of the further tumor manifestation [45]. This finding clearly indicates that both lymphomas arose from the same germinal center B cell and developed independently from each other into a Hodgkin's lymphoma and into follicular lymphoma.

MICROENVIRONMENT

Accumulating evidence supports the view that the tumor microenvironment might be more important for the clinical outcome of more non-Hodgkin's lymphomas than previously assumed. Recent genome-wide gene expression data provide evidence that this also holds true for classic Hodgkin's lymphoma [93]. In addition to genes probably expressed by the HRS cells (regulation of apoptosis and of cell cycle), the expression of molecules associated with immune response may have impact on the clinical outcome. Especially genes such as STAT1 (expressed by macrophages/monocytes) and LYZ and ALDH1A1 (macrophages) are described to be associated with poor outcome.

MOLECULES RELATED TO CLINICAL OUTCOME AND FOR THERAPEUTIC INTERVENTION

Classic Hodgkin's lymphoma is a curable disease in approximately 90% of the cases when aggressive chemotherapeutic drugs (ABVD, BEACOPP) are administered with or without combination with radiotherapy. Despite this success there are ongoing efforts to identify molecules that are able to select those patients refractory to current treatments or to allow alternative therapeutic approaches to circumvent highly aggressive drugs.

BCL-2, which is associated with prevention of apoptosis, is expressed in approximately 25% of the classic Hodgkin's lymphoma cases. Patients who have BCL-2–positive HRS cells display an only slightly worse overall survival. When combined with clinical risk factors, such as age (older than 45 years) and stage (III and IV), the expression of BCL-2 is a strong indicator for failure-free survival and overall survival [94].

Most recently the human germinal-center associated lymphoma (HGAL) gene has been found to be expressed in a proportion of classic Hodgkin's lymphoma cases. The expression of HGAL by the HRS cells not only confirms their germinal center derivation but also is linked to a tendency for better survival. Interestingly, a coexpression of HGAL and MUM1/IRF4 can be observed in most cases [95].

The impact of the number and type of tumor-infiltrating T cells on the clinical outcome or prognosis has been demonstrated for many malignancies. The analysis of the T-cell content and the T-cell composition present in classic Hodgkin's lymphoma cases revealed that a low infiltration by FOXP3-positive regulatory T cells in conjunction with a high number of TIA-1–positive cells identifies a patient group that is significantly associated with worse clinical outcome [96].

The composition of the tumor-infiltrating T cells and the expression of T-cell markers by the HRS cells itself seem to have an impact on the clinical course. Although the expression of these T-cell markers (CD3, CD4, CD8, CD45RO, TIA-1, and granzyme B) is also found in HRS cells carrying a B-cell genotype and is thus not lineage-specific; their presence is associated with a worse clinical outcome [97].

CD30, which is consistently expressed by the HRS cells, was often discussed as a therapeutic target for the treatment of classic Hodgkin's lymphoma. The treatment with anti-CD30 antibodies that were not coupled to radioactive molecules or other structures displayed only limited success [98]. This limited success is most likely because the CD30 signaling is disturbed in classic Hodgkin's lymphoma (Michael Hummel, PhD, unpublished data). CD30 is not only expressed by the HRS cells but may also occur in a soluble form (sCD30). Elevated serum levels of sCD30 (200 U/ml and more) in patients who have Hodgkin's lymphoma are associated with worse overall survival and failure-free survival [99].

Because constitutive NFκB overexpression is a common feature in classic Hodgkin's lymphoma that is demonstrated to be important for the survival of the HRS cells, blockage of NFκB activity by specific inhibitors seems to be an attractive therapeutic option. Previous attempts have been of limited success for unknown reasons.

Unexpectedly, the application of anti-CD20 antibodies (Rituximab) for the therapy of classic Hodgkin's lymphoma resulted in remission in a substantial number of patients, irrespective of the absence of CD20 on the HRS cells [100]. Because the CD20-treated number of classic Hodgkin's lymphoma patients is too small to draw final conclusions, larger patient cohorts have to be included and longer follow-up times are required to evaluate the suitability of this therapeutic approach.

References

[1] Hodgkin T. On some morbid appearances of the absorbent glands and spleen. Medical Chirurgical Transaction 1832;17:68–114.
[2] Wilks S. Cases of lardaceous disease and some allied affections, with remark. Guys Hosp Rep 1856;17:103–32.
[3] Wilks S. Cases with enlargement of the lymphatic glands and spleen (or Hodgkin's disease), with remarks. Guys Hospital Reports 1865;11:57.
[4] Wunderlich CA. Zwei Fälle von progressiven multiplen Lymphdrüsenhypertrophien. Archiv für physiologische Heilkunde 1858;12:122–31.
[5] Trousseau A. De l'adénie. Clin méd l'Hotel-Dieu Paris 1865;3:874–5.
[6] Langhans T. Das maligne lymphosarkom (pseudoleukämie). Virchow's Archiv f path Anatomie 1872;54:509–37.

[7] Greenfield WS. Specimens illustrative of the pathology of lymphadenoma and leucocythe-mia. Trans Path Soc London 1878;29:272–304.

[8] Sternberg C. Über eine eigenartige unter dem Bilde der Pseudoleukämie verlaufende Tuberculose des lymphatischen Apparates. Ztschr Heilk 1898;19:21–90.

[9] Reed DM. On the pathological changes in Hodgkin's disease, with especial reference to its relation to tuberculosis. John Hopkins Hosp Rep 1902;10:133–96.

[10] Fox H. Remarks on the microscopical preparations made from some of the original tissue described by Thomas Hodgkin 1832. Ann Med Hist 1926;8:370–4.

[11] Jackson HL, Parker F. Hodgkin's disease and allied disorders. New York: Oxford University Press;1947.

[12] Lukes RJ, Butler JJ. The pathology and nomenclature of Hodgkin's disease. Cancer Res 1966;26:1063–83.

[13] Harris NL, Jaffe ES, Stein H, et al. A revised European-American classification of lymphoid neoplasms: a proposal from the International Lymphoma Study Group. Blood 1994;84: 1361–92.

[14] Jaffe ES, Harris NL, Stein H, et al. Tumours of haematopoietic and lymphoid tissues. Lyon (France): IARCPress; 2001.

[15] Anagnostou D, Parker JW, Taylor CR, et al. Lacunar cells of nodular sclerosing Hodgkin's disease: an ultrastructural and immunohistologic study. Cancer 1977;39: 1032–43.

[16] Lorenzen J, Thiele J, Fischer R. The mummified Hodgkin cell: cell death in Hodgkin's disease. J Pathol 1997;182:288–98.

[17] Hess JL, Bodis S, Pinkus G, et al. Histopathologic grading of nodular sclerosis Hodgkin's disease. Lack of prognostic significance in 254 surgically staged patients. Cancer 1994;74:708–14.

[18] van Spronsen DJ, Vrints LW, Hofstra G, et al. Disappearance of prognostic significance of histopathological grading of nodular sclerosing Hodgkin's disease for unselected patients, 1972–92. Br J Haematol 1997;96:322–7.

[19] Diehl V, Sextro M, Franklin J, et al. Clinical presentation, course, and prognostic factors in lymphocyte-predominant Hodgkin's disease and lymphocyte-rich classical Hodgkin's disease: report from the European Task Force on Lymphoma Project on Lymphocyte-Predominant Hodgkin's Disease. J Clin Oncol 1999;17:776–83.

[20] Neiman RS, Rosen PJ, Lukes RJ. Lymphocyte-depletion Hodgkin's disease. A clinicopatho-logical entity. N Engl J Med 1973;288:751–5.

[21] Anagnostopoulos I, Hansmann ML, Franssila K, et al. European Task Force on lymphoma project on lymphocyte predominance Hodgkin disease: histologic and immunohistologic analysis of submitted cases reveals 2 types of Hodgkin disease with a nodular growth pattern and abundant lymphocytes. Blood 2000;96:1889–99.

[22] Stein H, Marafioti T, Foss HD, et al. Down-regulation of BOB.1/OBF.1 and Oct2 in classi-cal Hodgkin disease but not in lymphocyte predominant Hodgkin disease correlates with immunoglobulin transcription. Blood 2001;97:496–501.

[23] Marafioti T, Hummel M, Anagnostopoulos I, et al. Origin of nodular lymphocyte-predom-inant Hodgkin's disease from a clonal expansion of highly mutated germinal-center B cells. N Engl J Med 1997;337:453–8.

[24] Braeuninger A, Kuppers R, Strickler JG, et al. Hodgkin and Reed-Sternberg cells in lympho-cyte predominant Hodgkin disease represent clonal populations of germinal center-derived tumor B cells. Proc Natl Acad Sci U S A 1997;94:9337–42.

[25] Ohno T, Stribley JA, Wu G, et al. Clonality in nodular lymphocyte-predominant Hodgkin's disease. N Engl J Med 1997;337:459–65.

[26] Schwab U, Stein H, Gerdes J, et al. Production of a monoclonal antibody specific for Hodg-kin and Sternberg-Reed cells of Hodgkin's disease and a subset of normal lymphoid cells. Nature 1982;299:65–7.

[27] Pinkus GS, Thomas P, Said JW. Leu-M1—a marker for Reed-Sternberg cells in Hodgkin's disease. An immunoperoxidase study of paraffin-embedded tissues. Am J Pathol 1985;119:244–52.

[28] Olsson L. On the natural biology of the malignant cells in Hodgkin's disease. Int J Radiat Oncol Biol Phys 1985;11:37–48.

[29] Bargou RC, Mapara MY, Zugck C, et al. Characterization of a novel Hodgkin cell line, HD-MyZ, with myelomonocytic features mimicking Hodgkin's disease in severe combined immunodeficient mice. J Exp Med 1993;177:1257–68.

[30] Ree HJ, Khan AA, Qureshi MN, et al. Expression of cell adhesion molecules associated with germinal center in Hodgkin's disease: an immunohistochemical study. The germinal center related complex and histologic subtypes. Cancer 1994;73:1257–63.

[31] Strauchen JA, mitriu-Bona A. Immunopathology of Hodgkin's disease. Characterization of Reed-Sternberg cells with monoclonal antibodies. Am J Pathol 1986;123:293–300.

[32] Stein H, Mason DY, Gerdes J, et al. The expression of the Hodgkin's disease associated antigen Ki-1 in reactive and neoplastic lymphoid tissue: evidence that Reed-Sternberg cells and histiocytic malignancies are derived from activated lymphoid cells. Blood 1985;66: 848–58.

[33] Durkop H, Latza U, Hummel M, et al. Molecular cloning and expression of a new member of the nerve growth factor receptor family that is characteristic for Hodgkin's disease. Cell 1992;68:421–7.

[34] Gerdes J, Schwarting R, Stein H. High proliferative activity of Reed Sternberg associated antigen Ki-1 positive cells in normal lymphoid tissue. J Clin Pathol 1986;39:993–7.

[35] Tamaru J, Hummel M, Zemlin M, et al. Hodgkin's disease with a B-cell phenotype often shows a VDJ rearrangement and somatic mutations in the VH genes. Blood 1994;84:708–15.

[36] Kuppers R, Rajewsky K, Zhao M, et al. Hodgkin disease: Hodgkin and Reed-Sternberg cells picked from histological sections show clonal immunoglobulin gene rearrangements and appear to be derived from B cells at various stages of development. Proc Natl Acad Sci U S A 1994;91:10962–6.

[37] Hummel M, Marafioti T, Ziemann K, et al. Ig rearrangements in isolated Reed-Sternberg cells: conclusions from four different studies. Ann Oncol 1996;7(Suppl 4):31–3.

[38] Hummel M, Ziemann K, Lammert H, et al. Hodgkin's disease with monoclonal and polyclonal populations of Reed-Sternberg cells. N Engl J Med 1995;333:901–6.

[39] Marafioti T, Hummel M, Foss HD, et al. Hodgkin and Reed-Sternberg cells represent an expansion of a single clone originating from a germinal center B-cell with functional immunoglobulin gene rearrangements but defective immunoglobulin transcription. Blood 2000;95:1443–50.

[40] Seitz V, Hummel M, Marafioti T, et al. Detection of clonal T-cell receptor gamma-chain gene rearrangements in Reed-Sternberg cells of classic Hodgkin disease. Blood 2000;95: 3020–4.

[41] Muschen M, Rajewsky K, Brauninger A, et al. Rare occurrence of classical Hodgkin's disease as a T cell lymphoma. J Exp Med 2000;191:387–94.

[42] Kanzler H, Kuppers R, Hansmann ML, et al. Hodgkin and Reed-Sternberg cells in Hodgkin's disease represent the outgrowth of a dominant tumor clone derived from (crippled) germinal center B cells. J Exp Med 1996;184:1495–505.

[43] Ushmorov A, Ritz O, Hummel M, et al. Epigenetic silencing of the immunoglobulin heavy-chain gene in classical Hodgkin lymphoma-derived cell lines contributes to the loss of immunoglobulin expression. Blood 2004;104:3326–34.

[44] Ushmorov A, Leithauser F, Sakk O, et al. Epigenetic processes play a major role in B-cell-specific gene silencing in classical Hodgkin lymphoma. Blood 2006;107:2493–500.

[45] Marafioti T, Hummel M, Anagnostopoulos I, et al. Classical Hodgkin's disease and follicular lymphoma originating from the same germinal center B cell. J Clin Oncol 1999;17: 3804–9.

[46] Mathas S, Janz M, Hummel F, et al. Intrinsic inhibition of transcription factor E2A by HLH proteins ABF-1 and Id2 mediates reprogramming of neoplastic B cells in Hodgkin lymphoma. Nat Immunol 2006;7:207–15.

[47] Stein H, Hummel M, Durkop H, et al. Biology of Hodgkin's disease. In: Canellos GP, Lister TA, Sklar JL, editors. The lymphomas. Philadelphia: W.B. Saunders; 2007. p. 287–304.

[48] Foss HD, Reusch R, Demel G, et al. Frequent expression of the B-cell-specific activator protein in Reed-Sternberg cells of classical Hodgkin's disease provides further evidence for its B-cell origin. Blood 1999;94:3108–13.

[49] Hertel CB, Zhou XG, Hamilton-Dutoit SJ, et al. Loss of B cell identity correlates with loss of B cell-specific transcription factors in Hodgkin/Reed-Sternberg cells of classical Hodgkin lymphoma. Oncogene 2002;21:4908–20.

[50] Dallenbach FE, Stein H. Expression of T-cell-receptor beta chain in Reed-Sternberg cells. Lancet 1989;2:828–30.

[51] Kadin ME, Muramoto L, Said J. Expression of T-cell antigens on Reed-Sternberg cells in a subset of patients with nodular sclerosing and mixed cellularity Hodgkin's disease. Am J Pathol 1988;130:345–53.

[52] Krenacs L, Wellmann A, Sorbara L, et al. Cytotoxic cell antigen expression in anaplastic large cell lymphomas of T- and null-cell type and Hodgkin's disease: evidence for distinct cellular origin. Blood 1997;89:980–9.

[53] Oudejans JJ, Kummer JA, Jiwa M, et al. Granzyme B expression in Reed-Sternberg cells of Hodgkin's disease. Am J Pathol 1996;148:233–40.

[54] Drexler HG. Recent results on the biology of Hodgkin and Reed-Sternberg cells. I. Biopsy material. Leuk Lymphoma 1992;8:283–313.

[55] Pinkus GS, Pinkus JL, Langhoff E, et al. Fascin, a sensitive new marker for Reed-Sternberg cells of Hodgkin's disease. Evidence for a dendritic or B cell derivation? Am J Pathol 1997;150:543–62.

[56] Carbone A, Gloghini A, Volpe R, et al. Anti-vimentin antibody reactivity with Reed-Sternberg cells of Hodgkin's disease. Virchows Arch A Pathol Anat Histopathol 1990;417:43–8.

[57] Carbone A, Gloghini A, Aldinucci D, et al. Expression pattern of MUM1/IRF4 in the spectrum of pathology of Hodgkin's disease. Br J Haematol 2002;117:366–72.

[58] Falini B, Fizzotti M, Pucciarini A, et al. A monoclonal antibody (MUM1p) detects expression of the MUM1/IRF4 protein in a subset of germinal center B cells, plasma cells, and activated T cells. Blood 2000;95:2084–92.

[59] Bargou RC, Leng C, Krappmann D, et al. High-level nuclear NF-kappa B and Oct-2 is a common feature of cultured Hodgkin/Reed-Sternberg cells. Blood 1996;87:4340–7.

[60] Hatada EN, Krappmann D, Scheidereit C. NF-kappaB and the innate immune response. Curr Opin Immunol 2000;12:52–8.

[61] Krappmann D, Scheidereit C. Regulation of NF-kappa B activity by I kappa B alpha and I kappa B beta stability. Immunobiology 1997;198:3–13.

[62] Wood KM, Roff M, Hay RT. Defective IkappaBalpha in Hodgkin cell lines with constitutively active NF-kappaB. Oncogene 1998;16:2131–9.

[63] Emmerich F, Meiser M, Hummel M, et al. Overexpression of I kappa B alpha without inhibition of NF-kappaB activity and mutations in the I kappa B alpha gene in Reed-Sternberg cells. Blood 1999;94:3129–34.

[64] Cabannes E, Khan G, Aillet F, et al. Mutations in the IkBa gene in Hodgkin's disease suggest a tumour suppressor role for IkappaBalpha. Oncogene 1999;18:3063–70.

[65] Emmerich F, Theurich S, Hummel M, et al. Inactivating I kappa B epsilon mutations in Hodgkin/Reed-Sternberg cells. J Pathol 2003;201:413–20.

[66] Horie R, Watanabe T, Morishita Y, et al. Ligand-independent signaling by overexpressed CD30 drives NF-kappaB activation in Hodgkin-Reed-Sternberg cells. Oncogene 2002;21:2493–503.

[67] Annunziata CM, Safiran YJ, Irving SG, et al. Hodgkin disease: pharmacologic intervention of the CD40-NF kappa B pathway by a protease inhibitor. Blood 2000;96: 2841–8.

[68] Hinz M, Lemke P, Anagnostopoulos I, et al. Nuclear factor kappaB-dependent gene expression profiling of Hodgkin's disease tumor cells, pathogenetic significance, and link to constitutive signal transducer and activator of transcription 5a activity. J Exp Med 2002;196:605–17.

[69] Rodig SJ, Savage KJ, Nguyen V, et al. TRAF1 expression and c-Rel activation are useful adjuncts in distinguishing classical Hodgkin lymphoma from a subset of morphologically or immunophenotypically similar lymphomas. Am J Surg Pathol 2005;29: 196–203.

[70] Dukers DF, Meijer CJ, ten Berge RL, et al. High numbers of active caspase 3-positive Reed-Sternberg cells in pretreatment biopsy specimens of patients with Hodgkin disease predict favorable clinical outcome. Blood 2002;100:36–42.

[71] Tzankov A, Zimpfer A, Went P, et al. Aberrant expression of cell cycle regulators in Hodgkin and Reed-Sternberg cells of classical Hodgkin's lymphoma. Mod Pathol 2005;18: 90–6.

[72] Tzankov A, Zimpfer A, Lugli A, et al. High-throughput tissue microarray analysis of G1-cyclin alterations in classical Hodgkin's lymphoma indicates overexpression of cyclin E1. J Pathol 2003;199:201–7.

[73] Berglund M, Flordal E, Gullander J, et al. Molecular cytogenetic characterization of four commonly used cell lines derived from Hodgkin lymphoma. Cancer Genet Cytogenet 2003;141:43–8.

[74] Joos S, Kupper M, Ohl S, et al. Genomic imbalances including amplification of the tyrosine kinase gene JAK2 in CD30+ Hodgkin cells. Cancer Res 2000;60:549–52.

[75] Martin-Subero JI, Klapper W, Sotnikova A, et al. Chromosomal breakpoints affecting immunoglobulin loci are recurrent in Hodgkin and Reed-Sternberg cells of classical Hodgkin lymphoma. Cancer Res 2006;66:10332–8.

[76] Weiss LM, Strickler JG, Warnke RA, et al. Epstein-Barr viral DNA in tissues of Hodgkin's disease. Am J Pathol 1987;129:86–91.

[77] Herbst H, Niedobitek G, Kneba M, et al. High incidence of Epstein-Barr virus genomes in Hodgkin's disease. Am J Pathol 1990;137:13–8.

[78] Knecht H, Odermatt BF, Bachmann E, et al. Frequent detection of Epstein-Barr virus DNA by the polymerase chain reaction in lymph node biopsies from patients with Hodgkin's disease without genomic evidence of B- or T-cell clonality. Blood 1991;78:760–7.

[79] Hummel M, Anagnostopoulos I, Dallenbach F, et al. EBV infection patterns in Hodgkin's disease and normal lymphoid tissue: expression and cellular localization of EBV gene products. Br J Haematol 1992;82:689–94.

[80] Wu TC, Mann RB, Charache P, et al. Detection of EBV gene expression in Reed-Sternberg cells of Hodgkin's disease. Int J Cancer 1990;46:801–4.

[81] Herbst H. Epstein-Barr virus in Hodgkin's disease. Semin Cancer Biol 1996;7:183–9.

[82] Hummel M, Anagnostopoulos I, Korbjuhn P, et al. Epstein-Barr virus in B-cell non-Hodgkin's lymphomas: unexpected infection patterns and different infection incidence in low- and high-grade types. J Pathol 1995;175:263–71.

[83] Herbst H, Dallenbach F, Hummel M, et al. Epstein-Barr virus latent membrane protein expression in Hodgkin and Reed-Sternberg cells. Proc Natl Acad Sci U S A 1991;88: 4766–70.

[84] Bechtel D, Kurth J, Unkel C, et al. Transformation of BCR-deficient germinal-center B cells by EBV supports a major role of the virus in the pathogenesis of Hodgkin and posttransplantation lymphomas. Blood 2005;106:4345–50.

[85] Renne C, Willenbrock K, Kuppers R, et al. Autocrine- and paracrine-activated receptor tyrosine kinases in classic Hodgkin lymphoma. Blood 2005;105:4051–9.

[86] Renne C, Hinsch N, Willenbrock K, et al. The aberrant coexpression of several receptor tyrosine kinases is largely restricted to EBV-negative cases of classical Hodgkin's lymphoma. Int J Cancer 2007;120:2504–9.

[87] Abbondanzo SL, Sato N, Straus SE, et al. Acute infectious mononucleosis. CD30 (Ki-1) antigen expression and histologic correlations. Am J Clin Pathol 1990;93:698–702.

[88] Stein H, Johrens K, Anagnostopoulos I. Non-mediastinal grey zone lymphomas and report from the workshop. Eur J Haematol Suppl 2005;66:42–4.

[89] Banks PM. The distinction of Hodgkin's disease from T cell lymphoma. Semin Diagn Pathol 1992;9:279–83.

[90] Poppema S, Kluiver JL, Atayar C, et al. Report: workshop on mediastinal grey zone lymphoma. Eur J Haematol Suppl 2005;66:45–52.

[91] Ohno T, Smir BN, Weisenburger DD, et al. Origin of the Hodgkin/Reed-Sternberg cells in chronic lymphocytic leukemia with "Hodgkin's transformation". Blood 1998;91: 1757–61.

[92] Brauninger A, Hansmann ML, Strickler JG, et al. Identification of common germinal-center B-cell precursors in two patients with both Hodgkin's disease and non-Hodgkin's lymphoma. N Engl J Med 1999;340:1239–47.

[93] Sanchez-Aguilera A, Montalban C, de la CP, et al. Tumor microenvironment and mitotic checkpoint are key factors in the outcome of classic Hodgkin lymphoma. Blood 2006;108:662–8.

[94] Sup SJ, Alemany CA, Pohlman B, et al. Expression of bcl-2 in classical Hodgkin's lymphoma: an independent predictor of poor outcome. J Clin Oncol 2005;23:3773–9.

[95] Natkunam Y, Hsi ED, Aoun P, et al. Expression of the human germinal center-associated lymphoma (HGAL) protein identifies a subset of classic Hodgkin lymphoma of germinal center derivation and improved survival. Blood 2007;109:298–305.

[96] Alvaro T, Lejeune M, Salvado MT, et al. Outcome in Hodgkin's lymphoma can be predicted from the presence of accompanying cytotoxic and regulatory T cells. Clin Cancer Res 2005;11:1467–73.

[97] Asano N, Oshiro A, Matsuo K, et al. Prognostic significance of T-cell or cytotoxic molecules phenotype in classical Hodgkin's lymphoma: a clinicopathologic study. J Clin Oncol 2006;24:4626–33.

[98] Wahl AF, Klussman K, Thompson JD, et al. The anti-CD30 monoclonal antibody SGN-30 promotes growth arrest and DNA fragmentation in vitro and affects antitumor activity in models of Hodgkin's disease. Cancer Res 2002;62:3736–42.

[99] Visco C, Nadali G, Vassilakopoulos TP, et al. Very high levels of soluble CD30 recognize the patients with classical Hodgkin's lymphoma retaining a very poor prognosis. Eur J Haematol 2006;77:387–94.

[100] Younes A, Romaguera J, Hagemeister F, et al. A pilot study of rituximab in patients with recurrent, classic Hodgkin disease. Cancer 2003;98:310–4.

The Pathogenesis of Classical Hodgkin's Lymphoma: A Model for B-Cell Plasticity

Stephan Mathas, MD[a,b,*]

[a]Max-Delbrück-Center for Molecular Medicine, Robert-Rössle-Str. 10, 13125 Berlin, Germany
[b]Hematology, Oncology and Tumor Immunology, Charité, Medical University Berlin,
Campus Virchow-Klinikum, Campus Berlin-Buch, Augustenburger Platz 1,
13353 Berlin, Germany

THE PLASTICITY OF B-LYMPHOID CELLS

B-cell development is controlled by a complex network of transcription factors [1,2]. The B-cell lineage has been particularly informative for the analysis of lineage decision and commitment because its developmental stages are well defined. Key determinants of this transcription factor network are transcription factors PU.1, E2A, EBF, and Pax5, which act in a hierarchical and combinatorial manner to establish and to maintain the B cell–specific gene expression program. PU.1, E2A, and EBF are required for the generation of early B cells, whereas Pax5 has been proposed to act downstream of E2A and EBF and to be essential for commitment to the B-cell lineage and maintenance of the B-cell phenotype [2]. Inactivation of the E2A gene results in an early block of B-cell development, before immunoglobulin (Ig) rearrangement [3]. A similar phenotype has been described for EBF-deficient mice [4]. In the absence of Pax5, B-cell development is arrested at an early pro–B-cell stage in the bone marrow [2]. This regulatory network involves not only the sequential but also the concerted activity of these transcription factors, as exemplarily shown for regulation of the *mb-1* gene [5].

The targeted inactivation or enforced expression of these transcription factors in mouse models has not only demonstrated the importance of these transcriptional regulators for cell fate decisions, but has also revealed a remarkable degree of cellular plasticity in the hematopoietic system. Pax5-deficient B-cell progenitors thus retain a broad developmental potential, because they can differentiate under appropriate conditions into several hematopoietic lineages [6,7]. E2A-deficient bone marrow–derived cells show features of pro–B cells, but they also coexpress genes that are usually associated with other

*Max-Delbrück-Center for Molecular Medicine, Robert-Rössle-Str. 10, 13125 Berlin, Germany. E-mail address: stephan.mathas@charite.de

0889-8588/07/$ – see front matter
doi:10.1016/j.hoc.2007.06.016
© 2007 Elsevier Inc. All rights reserved.
hemonc.theclinics.com

hematopoietic lineages [8]. Similar to Pax5-deficient cells, E2A-deficient bone marrow cells reconstitute T, NK, myeloid, and other lineage cells, demonstrating that these cells possess properties of pluripotent progenitor cells [8]. A further example for the high plasticity of the B-cell compartment provides the observation that committed B cells can transdifferentiate into macrophages following enforced expression of C/EBP transcription factors [9]. These data have shown that cell fate specification in the hematopoietic system requires not only the activation of key factors that direct differentiation toward a specific lineage but also the concomitant suppression of alternative developmental pathways [10]. In differentiated B-lineage cells a balanced activity of lineage-instructive transcription factors and their regulators is thus required for maintenance of B-cell commitment. Following perturbation of this balanced activity, cells could acquire characteristics or even functional activities of other lineages, which has been referred to as reprogramming [11]. It is currently unclear whether such processes occur in the physiologic ontogenesis of B-lineage cells. In addition, such processes might occur during malignant transformation. Recent data suggest that reprogramming of B-lymphoid cells is involved in the pathogenesis of classical Hodgkin's lymphoma (HL).

THE ALTERED B-CELL TRANSCRIPTION FACTOR NETWORK IN HODGKIN'S AND REED-STERNBERG CELLS

The complexity of the B-cell maturation process predisposes this cell type to malignant transformation. Usually, B cell–derived lymphomas maintain the expression of B cell–associated genes. In rare cases, however, this expression program is lost. The most prominent example is HL. The malignant Hodgkin's/Reed-Sternberg (HRS) cells of HL derive from germinal center (GC) or post-GC B cells, which has been shown by the analysis of their rearranged and hypermutated immunoglobulin genes [12]. HRS cells do not display a B-cell phenotype, however, and their gene expression pattern does not allow an assignment to a defined hematopoietic lineage [13–17]. In particular, HRS cells have lost a considerable part of the B cell–specific gene expression pattern. This loss includes not only Ig/B cell–receptor (BCR) expression, but also components of the BCR complex (Ig-α/CD79A/mb-1; Ig-β/CD79B/ B29) and associated signaling molecules (eg, BLNK, Lck, Blk, and Lyn). In addition, HRS cells display a unique phenotype because they coexpress markers of different cell types. The investigation of transcription factors Oct-2, PU.1, or Bob.1/OBF, which are required for early B lymphocyte maturation [1], has revealed that all these transcription factors are not expressed in HRS cells [18,19]. In mice, activity of Oct-2, PU.1, or Bob.1/OBF is dispensable for maintenance of the B-cell commitment of mature B cells [1], suggesting that their loss is not necessarily involved in the down-regulation of B cell–specific genes in HRS cells. Apart from the loss of B cell–specific transcription factors, epigenetic alterations of B cell–specific genes have been described in HRS cells [20,21]. Epigenetic silencing of B cell–specific genes has been shown not only in HRS cell lines but also in single, microdissected primary HRS cells

[21]. In part, re-expression of some B cell–specific genes could be enforced by modulating epigenetic modification of HRS cell lines. It remains to be determined whether epigenetic silencing of B cell–specific genes is a primary or secondary event in HRS cells. The analysis of primary HRS cells has shown that some B cell–specific genes are not lacking in the whole tumor cell population, but expression is detectable in several cases, although in a low percentage of cells and at a low expression level [22,23]. These analyses suggest that the mechanism of inhibition of the B cell–specific gene expression program might be permissive and thus attributable to functional rather than structural defects.

A comprehensive analysis regarding the loss of B cell–specific gene expression results from the investigation of the B cell–determining transcription factors E2A, EBF, and Pax5. These transcription factors act in a hierarchical and combinatorial manner to establish and to maintain the B cell–specific gene expression program [2]. In contrast to the lost expression of their downstream target genes, expression of E2A, EBF, and Pax5 has been described in HRS cells [24–26]. Further analysis revealed a specifically altered DNA-binding activity of E2A in HRS cells [24]. This finding supports the hypothesis of a functional disruption of the B cell–specific transcription factor program in HRS cells. Comparative oligonucleotide microarray analyses of Hodgkin's and non-Hodgkin's cells revealed a specific overexpression of the E2A antagonists activated B-cell factor 1 (ABF-1) and inhibitor of differentiation 2 (Id2) in HRS cells [13,24,26]. ABF-1 can bind to E2A proteins and the resulting heterodimeric complexes can occupy E2A DNA binding sites (the so-called "E-box") [27]. Id2 lacks the basic region required for DNA binding [28]. Id2-E2A heterodimers therefore cannot bind to DNA, and Id2 indirectly inhibits E2A activity. In HRS cell lines, E2A-ABF-1 heterodimers were detectable, whereas, most probably because of the interaction with Id2, E2A homodimer activity was lacking [24]. These analyses indicated that the balance between E2A, Id2, and ABF-1 in HRS cells is shifted toward inactive E2A-ABF-1– and E2A-Id2–containing heterodimers [24,26]. In addition to ABF-1 and Id2, Notch1 might alter activity of transcription factors E2A, EBF, and Pax5 in HRS cells. Notch1 is overexpressed in HRS cells and supposed to be stimulated by Jagged1 [29]. Notch1 promotes degradation of E2A proteins and inhibits DNA binding of transcription factor EBF and transcription of the *Pax5* gene [30–32]. The functional significance of these data for the transcription factor network in HRS cells is currently not known.

The essential role of transcription factor E2A for expression of many B cell–specific genes has been recognized in different cellular systems [3]. ABF-1 and Id2 have been implicated in inhibition of E2A-dependent transcription [24,27,28]. Experimental support of this concept is provided by ectopic expression of ABF-1 and Id2 in non-Hodgkin's cells. Overexpression of Id proteins interferes with B- and T-lymphoid differentiation [33]. Furthermore, ABF-1 and Id2 are able to block expression of E2A-dependent B cell–specific genes, including Oct2, CD19, AID, CD79A, and EBF, which are all lacking in HRS cells [13,15,24]. In summary, in recent years great progress has been made in understanding the process of loss of B cell–specific gene expression in HRS cells. It can be assumed that these alterations are intimately linked to the process of malignant transformation. At least in a certain period during pathogenesis a strong activation of proliferative and antiapoptotic signaling pathways is required for the outgrowth of HRS cells, in particular to counteract the loss of BCR expression. These pathways are discussed in the following section.

DEREGULATED TRANSCRIPTION FACTORS IN HODGKIN'S LYMPHOMA WITH RESPECT TO PROLIFERATION AND SURVIVAL

Transcription factor nuclear factor kappa B (NF-κB) has been recognized as the transcription factor centrally involved in the orchestration of gene expression in HRS cells, in particular of genes involved in proliferation and apoptosis protection [34–37]. The mammalian NF-κB transcription factor family consists of the five NF-κB/Rel members RelA (p65), RelB, cRel, NF-κB1 (p50 and its precursor p105), and NF-κB2 (p52 and its precursor p100) [38,39]. These proteins can form dimers, which are in unstimulated cells retained in the cytoplasm by the inhibitor of NF-κB (IκB) proteins. The group of IκB proteins consists of IκBα, IκBβ, and IκBε, and the precursor proteins p100 and p105. Usually, the NF-κB pathway is triggered following stimulation by cytokines, chemokines, or microbial infection. In the classical NF-κB activation model, the inhibitor of NF-κB kinase (IKK) complex phosphorylates IκB proteins. Following phosphorylation, IκB proteins are targeted for proteasomal degradation, and liberated NF-κB dimers translocate into the nucleus, where NF-κB regulates transcription of various genes, including cytokines, chemokines, growth factors, adhesion molecules, and apoptosis regulators [40]. IκB proteins themselves are target genes of NF-κB, which establishes a negative feedback loop. In contrast to the usual transient NF-κB activation, aberrant constitutive activity of transcription factor NF-κB is a hallmark of HRS cells. In these cells, the classic NF-κB p50:p65 heterodimers can be found, but also cRel, RelB, and p52 are constitutively activated [34,35,41–43]. These data support the view that not only the classic but also the alternative NF-κB activation pathway is active in HRS cells. Constitutive NF-κB activity is required for proliferation and enhances apoptosis resistance of the HRS tumor cells [34,36,37]. Several functional and genomic alterations of the IKK/NF-κB pathway underline the importance of this system for HRS cells. First, in all investigated HRS cell lines the IKK complex is constitutively activated [42]. The significance of this finding for HRS cell biology is emphasized by the effects of pharmacologic inhibition of the IKK complex leading to cell death of HRS cells in vitro and in vivo [44]. The constitutive IKK activity argues for an ongoing upstream signaling activity, which might be delivered by signaling cascades induced by overexpressed TNF/death-receptor family members in HRS cells. CD30, CD40, RANK, and CD95 receptors are overexpressed on HRS cells, and stimulation of several of these receptors modifies NF-κB activity [45–49]. In particular, constitutively active CD30 signaling has been proposed to contribute to the NF-κB activity in HRS cells [50,51]. Second, deleterious mutations of the $I\kappa B\alpha$ and $I\kappa B\epsilon$ genes have been described in a significant number of HL cases [52–55]. As a result, nonfunctional or unstable $I\kappa B$ proteins are produced, and the negative NF-κB/$I\kappa$B feedback loop might be disrupted. Third, amplifications of the c-REL locus (2p14-15) with nuclear c-Rel protein accumulation are frequently found in HRS cells [41,56,57]. Finally, Bcl3, which shares structural similarity with $I\kappa$B proteins, is overexpressed in HRS cells and contributes to the activation of NF-κB by induction of NF-κB p50 homodimers [58]. Chromosomal gains and translocations of the $BCL3$ locus (19q13) indicate the importance of this finding for HRS cell biology [58–60]. Functional analyses revealed a central function of the constitutive NF-κB activity for HRS cell biology. Among NF-κB–regulated genes are cell cycle regulatory proteins, such as cyclin D2; antiapoptotic proteins, such as c-IAP2, Bcl-x_L, TRAF-1, and c-FLIP; cytokines, such as TNF-α, IL-13, IL-6, and GM-CSF; and cell surface receptors, such as CD40, CD86, or CCR7, all of them overexpressed in HRS cells [36,37,49]. The plethora of defects found in the NF-κB pathway points to the pressure on HRS cells to maintain high-level constitutive NF-κB activity and expression of the respective NF-κB target genes.

Similar to the constitutive NF-κB activity, constitutive aberrant expression of the AP-1 complex, containing c-Jun and JunB, is a pathogenetic hallmark of cHL [61,62]. AP-1 is composed of homo- or heterodimers formed by related Jun (c-Jun, JunB, JunD), Fos (c-Fos, FosB, Fra-1, Fra-2), and ATF family proteins, which might even act antagonistically [63,64]. Transcription of c-Jun and other AP-1 family members is rapidly and transiently stimulated by several extracellular signals. These trigger activation of the JNK, ERK1/2, or p38 MAP kinase pathways followed by AP-1 activation. With a specificity rarely documented for other oncogenes, constitutive c-Jun and JunB activity is found in the entire tumor cell population of all HL patients tested [61]. In cultured HL cells, c-Jun/AP-1 is up-regulated in a cell-autonomous manner, and AP-1 is required for proliferation of HRS cells. CD30 activation contributes to JunB overexpression in HRS cells [65], and MAPK activity might modulate AP-1 activation in primary HRS cells [66]. Constitutive JunB activity has been shown to stimulate expression of the TNF-receptor family member CD30, which is strongly overexpressed in HRS cells, and which itself might enforce activation of NF-κB and AP-1 in HRS cells [62,65]. Among the growing list of AP-1 target genes in HRS cells are the lymphocyte homing receptor CCR7, the cell cycle regulator cyclinD2, and the proto-oncogene c-met [61]. AP-1 is involved in the down-regulation of the B-cell phenotype by transcriptional activation of Id2 [24]. Furthermore, the CREB factor ATF-3 is selectively overexpressed in HRS cells and might interact with Jun proteins and enforce their transcriptional activity [67].

Another signaling pathway altered in HL is the Janus kinase/signal transducers and activators of transcription (JAK/STAT) signaling pathway. Similar to the $I\kappa$B/NF-κB signaling pathway, the JAK/STAT pathway is centrally involved in signaling cascades initiated by several cytokines [68]. These include

IL-5, IL-6, IL-9, IL-13, and GM-CSF, all described to be abundantly produced by HRS cells [69]. Following activation of the JAK/STAT pathway, activated JAKs phosphorylate STAT molecules, which are located in the cytoplasm before their activation. Following phosphorylation, STAT proteins dimerize and translocate into the nucleus, where they activate transcription of their target genes. In HRS cells, nuclear accumulation of phosphorylated STAT3, STAT5, and STAT6 has been shown, indicating transcriptional activity [37,70,71], and STAT3 and STAT6 are involved in proliferation and apoptosis protection of HRS cells [72,73]. Although mechanisms leading to the activation of STAT3 and STAT5 are less clarified, the constitutive STAT6 activity in HRS cells has been linked to IL-13 stimulation [70,72]. Genomic alterations of the JAK/STAT system point to an important pathogenetic role of this signaling pathway for HRS cells. Genomic amplifications of the *JAK2* gene (9p24) and mutations of the JAK regulator *SOCS-1* were described in HL [56,74,75]. SOCS proteins down-regulate JAK activity and are themselves target genes of STAT transcription factors. The finding that *SOCS-1* mutations in HL are associated with nuclear STAT5 accumulation indicates a disruption of this negative feedback loop in HRS cells [74,76]. Because constitutively activated STAT proteins, particularly STAT3 and STAT5, have been implicated in the process of malignant transformation [77], it will be important to further clarify the role of the JAK/STAT pathway for HRS cells.

THE TRANSCRIPTION FACTOR NETWORK IN HODGKIN'S AND REED-STERNBERG CELLS

Among lymphomas, HRS cells display a unique up-regulation of transcription factors NF-κB, AP-1, and STAT family members. This finding reveals the requirement for activation of strong, cell-autonomous signaling pathways for proliferation and apoptosis protection. It can be assumed that these transcription factors cooperate to enforce expression of not only cell cycle regulators and antiapoptotic proteins but also the unique expression of cytokines and chemokines (Fig. 1). Evidence has been presented for a crosstalk between these signaling pathways, in particular the NF-κB and the AP-1 pathways. First, a transcriptional cooperation of NF-κB and AP-1 has exemplarily been shown for cyclin D2 and the lymphocyte homing receptor CCR7 [61], both sharing NF-κB and AP-1 DNA binding sites in their promoter regions. The contribution of these transcription factors to transcriptional activation of, for example, GM-CSF, RANTES, or IL-6, all known to depend on NF-κB, AP-1, and STAT activity and to be overexpressed in HRS cells, has to be determined in future analysis. Second, NF-κB is involved in the regulation of the constitutively active JunB/AP-1 complex [61]. These data indicate that NF-κB does have an effect on the composition of the constitutively active AP-1 complex in HRS cells. In addition, NF-κB target genes were described to inhibit MAPK activity in different cell types. It remains to be determined whether constitutive NF-κB activity prevents MAPK activation in HRS cells. Third, following inhibition of NF-κB activity in HRS cell lines, a decrease of STAT5 activity has been

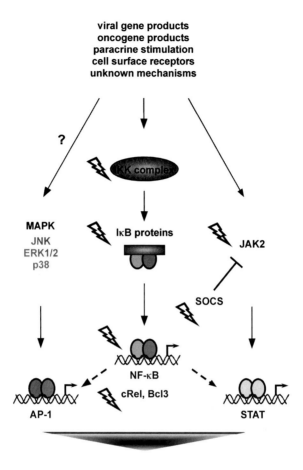

Fig. 1. Signaling pathways involved in proliferation, apoptosis protection, and aberrant gene expression of HRS cells. By different mechanisms (eg, activation of cell surface receptors or paracrine stimulation of HRS cells) the IKK/NF-κB, AP-1, and JAK/STAT signaling pathways are constitutively activated in HRS cells. In primary HRS cells, the activation status of MAPK is not entirely clear, indicated by "?". NF-κB has been shown to mediate in part activation of the AP-1 complex and to modulate STAT5 activity (dashed arrows indicate such a transcriptional crosstalk). The constitutive activation of these transcription factors results in part from a plethora of molecular and genomic defects in these signaling cascades (indicated by flashes; for details see text). The cooperative transcriptional activity of NF-κB, AP-1, and STAT transcription factors results in the unique gene expression pattern of, for example, antiapoptotic proteins, cytokines, and cell surface receptors of HRS cells.

observed [37]. These data indicate that constitutive NF-κB is a key player for HRS cell biology and orchestrates the integration of these signaling pathways regarding target gene activation.

THE REPROGRAMMING PROCESS OF HODGKIN'S AND REED-STERNBERG CELLS

HRS cells have lost the B-cell phenotype, including expression of the BCR [15]. Usually B cells with nonproductive Ig rearrangements or lack of BCR expression are prone to die by apoptosis in the process of the GC reaction. Obviously, HRS cells do not undergo apoptosis but instead expand to form HL. The need to strongly counteract apoptotic signals in a certain period during pathogenesis might deliver the explanation for the strong cell-autonomous activation of proliferative and antiapoptotic signaling pathways as reflected by the plethora of genomic defects discussed earlier. It has been postulated, however, that HRS cells require BCR-equivalent signaling cascades to survive [78]. In EBV-positive HL, the EBV-encoded protein LMP2A might deliver such BCR-equivalent signaling [79,80]. Such a scenario presumes that these BCR-negative cells would still depend on signaling pathways equivalent to BCR activation. The recently discovered plasticity of mature B cells and data showing reprogramming of HRS cells favor an alternative scenario.

HRS cells do not home in the GC, although they are derived from GC B cells. Instead, they are predominantly located in the interfollicular zone of the lymph nodes [81]. Because in the GC survival of B cells depends strictly on BCR signaling, HRS cells thus have left the environment in which the loss of BCR expression would have most dramatic consequences. The B-lineage infidelity of HRS cells might indicate that, concomitant with the loss of BCR expression, HRS cells become independent of BCR or BCR-equivalent signaling pathways. Instead, they might profit from activation of non–B-lineage signaling pathways with respect to apoptosis protection and proliferation. In this scenario, reprogramming of HRS cells would not be an epiphenomenon, but instead a key event in the process of malignant transformation.

Previous studies, particularly in mice, have shown that B-cell commitment can be reversed by disruption of the B cell–specific transcription factor program [7–9,82,83]. These models revealed that cell fate specification in the hematopoietic system requires not only activation of key factors that direct differentiation toward a specific lineage but also the concomitant suppression of alternative developmental pathways [10,11]. The degree of plasticity in the hematopoietic system has been particularly well documented from targeted inactivation of Pax5 and E2A and from enforced expression of C/EBP transcription factor in mice. These data have allowed for a better understanding of these processes during hematopoiesis. In mice lacking Pax5, early B-cell differentiation is blocked [84]. In addition, Pax5-deficient progenitor cells can differentiate into several hematopoietic lineages, including differentiation into T cells and myeloid cells [7]. This process is mediated in part by Pax5-mediated repression of *Notch1*, a key player for T-cell differentiation, or *CSF1R*, which is centrally involved in myeloid differentiation [85,86]. *Pax5* inactivation thus allows for promiscuous expression of non–B-lineage genes. These data support the view that lineage restriction is ensured by activation of lineage-specific genes concomitant with suppression of lineage-inappropriate ones [87]. A similar model has been proposed for transcription factor E2A [8]. Although inactivation of *E2A* results in a block of early B-cell development [88], E2A-deficient bone marrow–derived cells show a low-level expression of B lineage–specific genes. Similar to observations in Pax5-deficient progenitor cells, these E2A-deficient cells coexpress genes usually suppressed in B-lineage cells, among these *Gata3* and *Tcf7* (associated with T cells), *Gata1* and *Epor* (associated with erythroid cells), and *Csf3r* and *Csf1r* (associated with myeloid cells) [8]. This gene expression pattern resembles that observed in pluri- or multipotent progenitor cells, because hematopoietic multipotent progenitor cells exhibit a low level of multilineage gene expression (the so-called "transcriptional priming") [89]. E2A-deficient progenitor cells share not only the gene expression pattern but also functional properties with pluri- or multipotent progenitor cells [8]. In addition, by enforced expression of C/EBPα and C/EBPβ in differentiated B cells expression of B cell–specific genes is lost, and a myeloid cell-specific gene expression program becomes activated [9]. These data have shown that differentiated B cells can be reprogrammed into macrophages, which again points to the high degree of plasticity in the hematopoietic system. All these data indicate that B-cell commitment can be reversed by disruption of the B cell–specific transcription factor program. The loss or lineage-inappropriate expression of lineage-specific transcription factors in mice predisposes such cells for lymphoma development [90–92]. It is currently unclear whether similar processes occur during malignant transformation of human B cells.

What are the indications for a reprogramming process in HRS cells? Regarding the B cell–specific transcription factor program in HRS cells, PU.1, Oct-2, EBF, and Pax5 expression is reduced or lost, and E2A activity is functionally disrupted by overexpression of its antagonists ABF-1 and Id2 [18,19,24,93]. The function of the B cell–specific transcription factor program is thus disrupted in HRS cells. In accordance with this finding, the expression of B cell–specific genes, most of which are regulated in a hierarchical and combinatorial manner by EBF, E2A, and Pax5, has been lost [15]. As shown for E2A-deficient progenitor cells in mice, however, the expression of various B cell–specific markers (eg, CD19, CD20, CD79A) is not lacking completely, but can be detected in a varying proportion of HL cases, although in a low percentage of cells and at low expression level [22,23]. Concomitant with the loss or profound down-regulation of B cell–specific genes, HRS cells have been reported to express several non–B-lineage genes. Among these, expression of dendritic cell markers, transcription factors associated with T cells (GATA3, TCF1, T-bet), or macrophage-specific genes (eg, the CSF-1 receptor) has been shown in HRS cells [14,16,17,24]. All these genes are usually repressed in B cells by B cell–specific transcription factors [8,87]. In line with these data, reconstitution of E2A activity in HRS cells suppresses expression of B lineage–inappropriate genes [24].

Similarly, down-regulation of ABF-1 resulted in down-regulation of these genes, indicating a direct role of ABF-1 not only in extinction of B cell–specific gene expression but also in the up-regulation of B lineage–inappropriate genes [24]. Notch-1 expression and the NF-κB and AP-1–driven expression of cytokines, which are important for the differentiation of T-lineage cells, might facilitate up-regulation of these genes in HRS cells. Once up-regulated, these B lineage–inappropriate genes could themselves enforce the reprogramming process, because their ectopic expression in B cells can induce lineage switching. Together, in HRS cells the coexpression of genes specific for different hematopoietic lineages is reminiscent of the gene expression pattern in early pluripotent hematopoietic progenitor cells [89].

DO HODGKIN'S AND REED-STERNBERG CELLS REGAIN ASPECTS OF EARLY HEMATOPOIETIC PROGENITOR CELLS?

In mouse models committed B cells can be reprogrammed into cells with multi-lineage potential, which is a key property of hematopoietic stem cells (HSC) or early hematopoietic progenitor cells. Although the phenotypic and functional properties of HSC or early progenitor cells have been studied extensively, pathways involved in the process of stem cell maintenance or renewal of early progenitors are only defined in part. These pathways must allow for proliferation while they suppress differentiation or induction of apoptosis. In recent years, several signaling pathways required for the maintenance of early progenitor self-renewal and of an undifferentiated cellular state have been identified [94]. These pathways can be classified as cell-intrinsic or, if they result from an interaction with the cellular microenvironment, cell-extrinsic. Well-characterized cell-intrinsic factors for hematopoietic progenitor cell self-renewal include transcription factor STAT5 [95], the zinc-finger transcription factor GATA-2 [96,97], factors of the homeobox (Hox) gene family [98], and the Zinc-finger repressor growth factor independence 1 (Gfi1) [99]. For all these factors it has been shown in vivo that modulation of their activity severely alters HSC or early progenitor self-renewal capacity. Constitutive activation of several of these factors in the HSC compartment results in a dramatic expansion of multipotent progenitor cells in vitro and in vivo. In addition, a central role in the process of HSC self-renewal has been attributed to the Polycomb group (PcG) proteins. Members of this group have been shown not only to enhance the expansion of the stem cell pool but also to suppress genes involved in the process of cellular differentiation. Among these genes are factors that promote lineage specification, cell death, or cell cycle arrest. In particular Bmi1, a member of the Polycomb repression complex 1 (PRC1), enhances expansion of multipotent progenitor cells, and is itself involved in the regulation of Hox genes [100,101]. Apart from these cell-intrinsic factors, several cell-extrinsic regulators, resulting from stimulation of HSC or multipotent progenitor cells from the microenvironment, have been identified [94]. First, the highly conserved Notch signaling pathway has been recognized as master regulator of cell fate decisions. Notch signaling is highly activated in HSC and is down-regulated following differentiation [102]. Furthermore, enforced activation of Notch signaling induces an expansion of the HSC pool and inhibits differentiation. Second, the Wnt pathway regulates HSC self-renewal. Enhanced LEF1/TCF (lymphoid enhancer binding factor 1; T cell–specific factor) activity has thus been reported in HSC, and inhibition of the Wnt pathway reduces expansion of the HSC compartment and reconstitution of hematopoiesis in vivo [103]. In addition to these briefly discussed pathways, altered expression of cell cycle regulators, such as p21, transcription factor dosage effects (as shown for PU.1 and GATA factors), and the family of Hedgehog (Hh) proteins are important for HSC or multipotent hematopoietic progenitor cell biology [94].

There is increasing experimental support that HRS share signaling pathways involved in the biology of early hematopoietic progenitor cells. HRS cells exhibit gene expression of multiple hematopoietic lineages, which is reminiscent of the low-level multilineage gene expression found in hematopoietic multipotent progenitors. Several of the intrinsic and extrinsic pathways important for the self-renewal of HSC or multipotent progenitor cells have been described to be among lymphomas specifically altered in HRS cells of HL. First, the GATA transcription factor GATA-2 was found specifically overexpressed in HRS cells [104]. In contrast, GATA-2 was not expressed in normal GC B cells or other B cell–derived lymphomas. As enforced expression of GATA-2 in pluripotent hematopoietic cells blocks differentiation and has been implicated in maintenance of a progenitor cell status, GATA-2 might be involved in the reprogramming process of HRS cells. Second, strong expression of Notch1 and Notch2 surface receptors has been identified in HRS cells [29,105]. In particular, the Notch1 pathway is supposed to be activated on HRS cells by Jagged1 and mediates proliferation and apoptosis resistance. The aberrant Notch activation in B cell–derived HRS cells might be seen as expression of a B lineage–inappropriate, T cell–associated gene. Indeed, in other cellular systems, Notch1 induces degradation of E2A proteins, inhibits EBF DNA binding, and promotes T cell development while concomitantly suppressing B cell development [30–32]. Apart from being seen as a lineage-inappropriate, T cell–associated gene in B cell–derived HRS cells, Notch1 overexpression might reflect their early progenitor state. Furthermore, in such cells Notch positively regulates GATA-2, which might explain GATA-2 expression in HRS cells [106]. Third, HRS cells express proteins of the PcG complexes, including Bmi1 [107,108]. Expression of these genes could not be identified in normal mature B cells or other B cell–derived lymphomas, and is again reminiscent to the expression pattern in early hematopoietic progenitor cells. In addition to activation of these genes, selective overexpression of members of the Hox gene cluster has been shown in HRS cells [109]. Down-regulation of the Hox gene HoxB9 resulted in proliferation arrest of the HRS cells. Furthermore, activation of the JAK/STAT pathway, in particular STAT5, has been described in HRS cell lines and primary cells [37,74]. Although for several of these genes and pathways their impact on lineage-specific gene silencing, loss of cell identity, or maintenance of an undifferentiated cellular stage is currently unclear, the altered expression of these genes might explain the unique phenotype of HRS cells. In HRS cells, the unique expression pattern of genes usually expressed at and restricted to an early progenitor cell stage might be the final result of the reprogramming process from the GC B cell to a cell resembling an undifferentiated hematopoietic progenitor cell (Fig. 2).

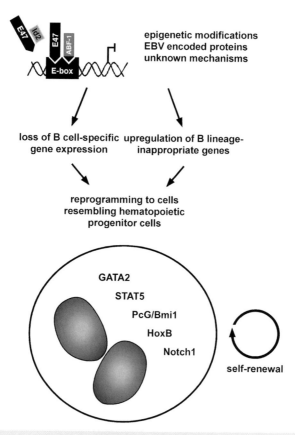

Fig. 2. Consequences of the deregulated activity of B cell–specific transcription factors in HL. In HRS cells of HL the activity of the B cell–determining transcription factor E2A is functionally disrupted by overexpression of its antagonists ABF-1 and Id2. Furthermore, by EBV-encoded proteins (eg, LMP2A) and as yet unknown mechanisms the expression of B cell–specific genes is lost. The loss of the B cell–specific gene expression program allows for up-regulation of usually suppressed, B lineage–inappropriate genes. As a result, HRS cells exhibit a gene expression pattern of multiple hematopoietic lineages, which is reminiscent of the low-level multilineage gene expression observed in hematopoietic multipotent progenitor cells. Finally, HRS cells show a specific overexpression of factors involved in the proliferation and expansion of early hematopoietic progenitors and in the maintenance of an undifferentiated cellular stage (eg, STAT5, Notch1, GATA-2, HoxB, Bmi1). These processes might support the self-renewal of HRS tumor cells.

SUMMARY

It has been shown in particular in mouse models that committed B-lymphoid cells are able to regain multilineage potential and to transdifferentiate into non–B-lineage cells. This process of lineage switching has been referred to as reprogramming. These data have revealed that adhesion to the B-lineage pathway depends on the balanced activity of lineage-instructive transcription factors and their regulators. These models have challenged the previous rigid view of cellular differentiation and revealed a remarkable degree of cellular plasticity in the hematopoietic system. It is currently unclear whether similar processes occur in vivo during the physiologic process of B-cell ontogenesis or during the process of malignant transformation of B cells. Such lineage infidelity might occur in an exceptional context, in particular in that of major alterations of the physiologic cellular equilibrium (eg, during the course of malignant transformation). Importantly, lymphoid cells in mice are prone to lymphoma development following loss of lineage-specific transcription factors or lineage-inappropriate expression of such factors. These observations suggest that a disruption of the lineage-specific transcription factor program in lymphoid cells might be linked to the process of malignant transformation.

There is increasing experimental evidence that HL can serve as a model for these processes in human B-lymphoid cells. HRS cells derive from GC B cells. They have lost the B cell–specific gene expression program and, in contrast, show simultaneous expression of genes associated with non–B-lineage cells. This expression pattern is reminiscent of that observed in multipotent progenitor cells. In addition, HRS cells show a unique expression of genes required for maintenance of the hematopoietic early progenitor cell fate. It might be assumed that HRS cells are reprogrammed to cells resembling undifferentiated hematopoietic progenitor cells. HL is thus a unique example to demonstrate the plasticity of human lymphoid cells. The further understanding of the reprogramming process might allow for the development of new treatment strategies for HL patients.

Acknowledgments

I thank Bernd Dörken for his generous support of my work, and Martin Janz and Andreas Lietz for critical reading of the manuscript. I apologize to colleagues whose articles could not be cited because of space limitations. Work of the author described in this article was supported in part by grants from the Deutsche Forschungsgemeinschaft, the Berliner Krebsgesellschaft, the Deutsche Krebshilfe, and the National Genome Research Network.

References

[1] Matthias P, Rolink AG. Transcriptional networks in developing and mature B cells. Nat Rev Immunol 2005;5(6):497–508.
[2] Busslinger M. Transcriptional control of early B cell development. Annu Rev Immunol 2004;22:55–79.
[3] Kee BL, Quong MW, Murre C. E2A proteins: essential regulators at multiple stages of B-cell development. Immunol Rev 2000;175:138–49.

[4] Lin H, Grosschedl R. Failure of B-cell differentiation in mice lacking the transcription factor EBF. Nature 1995;376(6537):263–7.

[5] Sigvardsson M, Clark DR, Fitzsimmons D, et al. Early B-cell factor, E2A, and Pax-5 cooperate to activate the early B cell-specific mb-1 promoter. Mol Cell Biol 2002;22(24): 8539–51.

[6] Nutt SL, Eberhard D, Horcher M, et al. Pax5 determines the identity of B cells from the beginning to the end of B-lymphopoiesis. Int Rev Immunol 2001;20(1):65–82.

[7] Rolink AG, Schaniel C, Bruno L, et al. In vitro and in vivo plasticity of Pax5-deficient pre-B I cells. Immunol Lett 2002;82(1–2):35–40.

[8] Ikawa T, Kawamoto H, Wright LY, et al. Long-term cultured E2A-deficient hematopoietic progenitor cells are pluripotent. Immunity 2004;20(3):349–60.

[9] Xie H, Ye M, Feng R, et al. Stepwise reprogramming of B cells into macrophages. Cell 2004;117(5):663–76.

[10] Laiosa CV, Stadtfeld M, Graf T. Determinants of lymphoid-myeloid lineage diversification. Annu Rev Immunol 2006;24:705–38.

[11] Graf T. Differentiation plasticity of hematopoietic cells. Blood 2002;99(9):3089–101.

[12] Küppers R, Rajewsky K. The origin of Hodgkin and Reed/Sternberg cells in Hodgkin's disease. Annu Rev Immunol 1998;16:471–93.

[13] Küppers R, Klein U, Schwering I, et al. Identification of Hodgkin and Reed-Sternberg cell-specific genes by gene expression profiling. J Clin Invest 2003;111(4):529–37.

[14] Pileri SA, Ascani S, Leoncini L, et al. Hodgkin's lymphoma: the pathologist's viewpoint. J Clin Pathol 2002;55(3):162–76.

[15] Schwering I, Bräuninger A, Klein U, et al. Loss of the B-lineage-specific gene expression program in Hodgkin and Reed-Sternberg cells of Hodgkin's lymphoma. Blood 2003; 101(4):1505–12.

[16] Dorfman DM, Hwang ES, Shahsafaei A, et al. T-bet, a T cell-associated transcription factor, is expressed in Hodgkin's lymphoma. Hum Pathol 2005;36(1):10–5.

[17] Atayar C, Poppema S, Blokzijl T, et al. Expression of the T-cell transcription factors, GATA-3 and T-bet, in the neoplastic cells of Hodgkin's lymphomas. Am J Pathol 2005;166(1): 127–34.

[18] Jundt F, Kley K, Anagnostopoulos I, et al. Loss of PU.1 expression is associated with defective immunoglobulin transcription in Hodgkin and Reed-Sternberg cells of classical Hodgkin disease. Blood 2002;99(8):3060–2.

[19] Stein H, Marafioti T, Foss HD, et al. Down-regulation of BOB.1/OBF.1 and Oct2 in classical Hodgkin disease but not in lymphocyte predominant Hodgkin disease correlates with immunoglobulin transcription. Blood 2001;97(2):496–501.

[20] Ushmorov A, Ritz O, Hummel M, et al. Epigenetic silencing of the immunoglobulin heavy chain gene in classical Hodgkin's lymphoma-derived cell lines contributes to the loss of immunoglobulin expression. Blood 2004;104(10):3326–34.

[21] Ushmorov A, Leithäuser F, Sakk O, et al. Epigenetic processes play a major role in B-cell-specific gene silencing in classical Hodgkin's lymphoma. Blood 2006;107(6): 2493–500.

[22] Korkolopoulou P, Cordell J, Jones M, et al. The expression of the B-cell marker mb-1 (CD79a) in Hodgkin's disease. Histopathology 1994;24(6):511–5.

[23] Watanabe K, Yamashita Y, Nakayama A, et al. Varied B-cell immunophenotypes of Hodgkin/Reed-Sternberg cells in classic Hodgkin's disease. Histopathology 2000;36(4): 353–61.

[24] Mathas S, Janz M, Hummel F, et al. Intrinsic inhibition of transcription factor E2A by HLH proteins ABF-1 and Id2 mediates reprogramming of neoplastic B cells in Hodgkin's lymphoma. Nat Immunol 2006;7(2):207–15.

[25] Foss HD, Reusch R, Demel G, et al. Frequent expression of the B-cell-specific activator protein in Reed-Sternberg cells of classical Hodgkin's disease provides further evidence for its B-cell origin. Blood 1999;94(9):3108–13.

[26] Renne C, Martin-Subero JI, Eickernjager M, et al. Aberrant expression of ID2, a suppressor of B-cell-specific gene expression, in Hodgkin's lymphoma. Am J Pathol 2006;169(2): 655–64.

[27] Massari ME, Rivera RR, Voland JR, et al. Characterization of ABF-1, a novel basic helix-loop-helix transcription factor expressed in activated B lymphocytes. Mol Cell Biol 1998;18(6):3130–9.

[28] Rivera R, Murre C. The regulation and function of the Id proteins in lymphocyte development. Oncogene 2001;20(58):8308–16.

[29] Jundt F, Anagnostopoulos I, Förster R, et al. Activated Notch 1 signaling promotes tumor cell proliferation and survival in Hodgkin and anaplastic large cell lymphoma. Blood 2002;99(9):3398–403.

[30] Nie L, Xu M, Vladimirova A, et al. Notch-induced E2A ubiquitination and degradation are controlled by MAP kinase activities. EMBO J 2003;22(21):5780–92.

[31] Smith EM, Akerblad P, Kadesch T, et al. Inhibition of EBF function by active Notch signaling reveals a novel regulatory pathway in early B-cell development. Blood 2005;106(6): 1995–2001.

[32] Pui JC, Allman D, Xu L, et al. Notch 1 expression in early lymphopoiesis influences B versus T lineage determination. Immunity 1999;11(3):299–308.

[33] Sun XH. Constitutive expression of the Id1 gene impairs mouse B cell development. Cell 1994;79(5):893–900.

[34] Bargou RC, Emmerich F, Krappmann D, et al. Constitutive nuclear factor-kappaB-RelA activation is required for proliferation and survival of Hodgkin's disease tumor cells. J Clin Invest 1997;100(12):2961–9.

[35] Bargou RC, Leng C, Krappmann D, et al. High-level nuclear NF-kappa B and Oct-2 is a common feature of cultured Hodgkin/Reed-Sternberg cells. Blood 1996;87(10):4340–7.

[36] Hinz M, Löser P, Mathas S, et al. Constitutive NF-kappaB maintains high expression of a characteristic gene network, including CD40, CD86, and a set of antiapoptotic genes in Hodgkin/Reed-Sternberg cells. Blood 2001;97(9):2798–807.

[37] Hinz M, Lemke P, Anagnostopoulos I, et al. Nuclear factor kappaB-dependent gene expression profiling of Hodgkin's disease tumor cells, pathogenetic significance, and link to constitutive signal transducer and activator of transcription 5a activity. J Exp Med 2002;196(5):605–17.

[38] Luo JL, Kamata H, Karin M. IKK/NF-kappaB signaling: balancing life and death—a new approach to cancer therapy. J Clin Invest 2005;115(10):2625–32.

[39] Bonizzi G, Karin M. The two NF-kappaB activation pathways and their role in innate and adaptive immunity. Trends Immunol 2004;25(6):280–8.

[40] Karin M, Ben-Neriah Y. Phosphorylation meets ubiquitination: the control of NF-[kappa]B activity. Annu Rev Immunol 2000;18:621–63.

[41] Barth TF, Martin-Subero JI, Joos S, et al. Gains of 2p involving the REL locus correlate with nuclear c-Rel protein accumulation in neoplastic cells of classical Hodgkin's lymphoma. Blood 2003;101(9):3681–6.

[42] Krappmann D, Emmerich F, Kordes U, et al. Molecular mechanisms of constitutive NF-kappaB/Rel activation in Hodgkin/Reed-Sternberg cells. Oncogene 1999;18(4):943–53.

[43] Nonaka M, Horie R, Itoh K, et al. Aberrant NF-kappaB2/p52 expression in Hodgkin/Reed-Sternberg cells and CD30-transformed rat fibroblasts. Oncogene 2005;24(24): 3976–86.

[44] Mathas S, Lietz A, Janz M, et al. Inhibition of NF-kappaB essentially contributes to arsenic-induced apoptosis. Blood 2003;102(3):1028–34.

[45] Fiumara P, Snell V, Li Y, et al. Functional expression of receptor activator of nuclear factor kappaB in Hodgkin disease cell lines. Blood 2001;98(9):2784–90.

[46] Dürkop H, Latza U, Hummel M, et al. Molecular cloning and expression of a new member of the nerve growth factor receptor family that is characteristic for Hodgkin's disease. Cell 1992;68(3):421–7.

[47] Annunziata CM, Safiran YJ, Irving SG, et al. Hodgkin disease: pharmacologic intervention of the CD40-NF kappa B pathway by a protease inhibitor. Blood 2000;96(8): 2841–8.

[48] Carbone A, Gloghini A, Gattei V, et al. Expression of functional CD40 antigen on Reed-Sternberg cells and Hodgkin's disease cell lines. Blood 1995;85(3): 780–9.

[49] Mathas S, Lietz A, Anagnostopoulos I, et al. c-FLIP mediates resistance of Hodgkin/Reed-Sternberg cells to death receptor-induced apoptosis. J Exp Med 2004;199(8): 1041–52.

[50] Horie R, Watanabe T, Ito K, et al. Cytoplasmic aggregation of TRAF2 and TRAF5 proteins in the Hodgkin-Reed-Sternberg cells. Am J Pathol 2002;160(5):1647–54.

[51] Horie R, Watanabe T, Morishita Y, et al. Ligand-independent signaling by overexpressed CD30 drives NF-kappaB activation in Hodgkin-Reed-Sternberg cells. Oncogene 2002; 21(16):2493–503.

[52] Emmerich F, Theurich S, Hummel M, et al. Inactivating I kappa B epsilon mutations in Hodgkin/Reed-Sternberg cells. J Pathol 2003;201(3):413–20.

[53] Emmerich F, Meiser M, Hummel M, et al. Overexpression of I kappa B alpha without inhibition of NF-kappaB activity and mutations in the I kappa B alpha gene in Reed-Sternberg cells. Blood 1999;94(9):3129–34.

[54] Wood KM, Roff M, Hay RT. Defective IkappaBalpha in Hodgkin cell lines with constitutively active NF-kappaB. Oncogene 1998;16(16):2131–9.

[55] Jungnickel B, Staratschek-Jox A, Bräuninger A, et al. Clonal deleterious mutations in the IkappaBalpha gene in the malignant cells in Hodgkin's lymphoma. J Exp Med 2000; 191(2):395–402.

[56] Joos S, Granzow M, Holtgreve-Grez H, et al. Hodgkin's lymphoma cell lines are characterized by frequent aberrations on chromosomes 2p and 9p including REL and JAK2. Int J Cancer 2003;103(4):489–95.

[57] Martin-Subero JI, Gesk S, Harder L, et al. Recurrent involvement of the REL and BCL11A loci in classical Hodgkin's lymphoma. Blood 2002;99(4):1474–7.

[58] Mathas S, Jöhrens K, Joos S, et al. Elevated NF-kappaB p50 complex formation and Bcl-3 expression in classical Hodgkin, anaplastic large-cell, and other peripheral T-cell lymphomas. Blood 2005;106(13):4287–93.

[59] Martin-Subero JI, Klapper W, Sotnikova A, et al. Chromosomal breakpoints affecting immunoglobulin loci are recurrent in Hodgkin and Reed-Sternberg cells of classical Hodgkin's lymphoma. Cancer Res 2006;66(21):10332–8.

[60] Martin-Subero JI, Wlodarska I, Bastard C, et al. Chromosomal rearrangements involving the BCL3 locus are recurrent in classical Hodgkin and peripheral T-cell lymphoma. Blood 2006;108(1):401–2, author reply 402–3.

[61] Mathas S, Hinz M, Anagnostopoulos I, et al. Aberrantly expressed c-Jun and JunB are a hallmark of Hodgkin's lymphoma cells, stimulate proliferation and synergize with NF-kappa B. EMBO J 2002;21(15):4104–13.

[62] Watanabe M, Ogawa Y, Ito K, et al. AP-1 mediated relief of repressive activity of the CD30 promoter microsatellite in Hodgkin and Reed-Sternberg cells. Am J Pathol 2003;163(2): 633–41.

[63] Shaulian E, Karin M. AP-1 as a regulator of cell life and death. Nat Cell Biol 2002;4(5): E131–6.

[64] Szabowski A, Maas-Szabowski N, Andrecht S, et al. c-Jun and JunB antagonistically control cytokine-regulated mesenchymal-epidermal interaction in skin. Cell 2000;103(5): 745–55.

[65] Watanabe M, Sasaki M, Itoh K, et al. JunB induced by constitutive CD30-extracellular signal-regulated kinase 1/2 mitogen-activated protein kinase signaling activates the CD30 promoter in anaplastic large cell lymphoma and Reed-Sternberg cells of Hodgkin's lymphoma. Cancer Res 2005;65(17):7628–34.

[66] Zheng B, Fiumara P, Li YV, et al. MEK/ERK pathway is aberrantly active in Hodgkin disease: a signaling pathway shared by CD30, CD40, and RANK that regulates cell proliferation and survival. Blood 2003;102(3):1019–27.

[67] Janz M, Hummel M, Truss M, et al. Classical Hodgkin's lymphoma is characterized by high constitutive expression of activating transcription factor 3 (ATF3), which promotes viability of Hodgkin/Reed-Sternberg cells. Blood 2006;107(6):2536–9.

[68] Shuai K, Liu B. Regulation of JAK-STAT signalling in the immune system. Nat Rev Immunol 2003;3(11):900–11.

[69] Skinnider BF, Mak TW. The role of cytokines in classical Hodgkin's lymphoma. Blood 2002;99(12):4283–97.

[70] Skinnider BF, Elia AJ, Gascoyne RD, et al. Signal transducer and activator of transcription 6 is frequently activated in Hodgkin and Reed-Sternberg cells of Hodgkin's lymphoma. Blood 2002;99(2):618–26.

[71] Kube D, Holtick U, Vockerodt M, et al. STAT3 is constitutively activated in Hodgkin cell lines. Blood 2001;98(3):762–70.

[72] Trieu Y, Wen XY, Skinnider BF, et al. Soluble interleukin-13Ralpha2 decoy receptor inhibits Hodgkin's lymphoma growth in vitro and in vivo. Cancer Res 2004;64(9):3271–5.

[73] Holtick U, Vockerodt M, Pinkert D, et al. STAT3 is essential for Hodgkin's lymphoma cell proliferation and is a target of tyrphostin AG17 which confers sensitization for apoptosis. Leukemia 2005;19(6):936–44.

[74] Weniger MA, Melzner I, Menz CK, et al. Mutations of the tumor suppressor gene SOCS-1 in classical Hodgkin's lymphoma are frequent and associated with nuclear phospho-STAT5 accumulation. Oncogene 2006;25(18):2679–84.

[75] Joos S, Küpper M, Ohl S, et al. Genomic imbalances including amplification of the tyrosine kinase gene JAK2 in CD30+ Hodgkin cells. Cancer Res 2000;60(3):549–52.

[76] Baus D, Pfitzner E. Specific function of STAT3, SOCS1, and SOCS3 in the regulation of proliferation and survival of classical Hodgkin's lymphoma cells. Int J Cancer 2006;118(6): 1404–13.

[77] Khwaja A. The role of Janus kinases in haemopoiesis and haematological malignancy. Br J Haematol 2006;134(4):366–84.

[78] Ambinder R. Infection and lymphoma. N Engl J Med 2003;349(14):1309–11.

[79] Caldwell RG, Wilson JB, Anderson SJ, et al. Epstein-Barr virus LMP2A drives B cell development and survival in the absence of normal B cell receptor signals. Immunity 1998;9(3):405–11.

[80] Chapman AL, Rickinson AB. Epstein-Barr virus in Hodgkin's disease. Ann Oncol 1998;9(Suppl 5):S5–16.

[81] Höpken UE, Foss HD, Meyer D, et al. Up-regulation of the chemokine receptor CCR7 in classical but not in lymphocyte-predominant Hodgkin disease correlates with distinct dissemination of neoplastic cells in lymphoid organs. Blood 2002;99(4):1109–16.

[82] Nutt SL, Heavey B, Rolink AG, et al. Commitment to the B-lymphoid lineage depends on the transcription factor Pax5. Nature 1999;401(6753):556–62.

[83] Mikkola I, Heavey B, Horcher M, et al. Reversion of B cell commitment upon loss of Pax5 expression. Science 2002;297(5578):110–3.

[84] Urbanek P, Wang ZQ, Fetka I, et al. Complete block of early B cell differentiation and altered patterning of the posterior midbrain in mice lacking Pax5/BSAP. Cell 1994; 79(5):901–12.

[85] Souabni A, Cobaleda C, Schebesta M, et al. Pax5 promotes B lymphopoiesis and blocks T cell development by repressing Notch1. Immunity 2002;17(6):781–93.

[86] Tagoh H, Ingram R, Wilson N, et al. The mechanism of repression of the myeloid-specific c-fms gene by Pax5 during B lineage restriction. EMBO J 2006;25(5):1070–80.

[87] Delogu A, Schebesta A, Sun Q, et al. Gene repression by Pax5 in B cells is essential for blood cell homeostasis and is reversed in plasma cells. Immunity 2006;24(3):269–81.

[88] Bain G, Maandag EC, Izon DJ, et al. E2A proteins are required for proper B cell development and initiation of immunoglobulin gene rearrangements. Cell 1994;79(5):885–92.

[89] Hu M, Krause D, Greaves M, et al. Multilineage gene expression precedes commitment in the hemopoietic system. Genes Dev 1997;11(6):774–85.

[90] Souabni A, Jochum W, Busslinger M. Oncogenic role of Pax5 in the T-lymphoid lineage upon ectopic expression from the immunoglobulin heavy-chain locus. Blood 2007; 109(1):281–9.

[91] Bain G, Engel I, Robanus Maandag EC, et al. E2A deficiency leads to abnormalities in alphabeta T-cell development and to rapid development of T-cell lymphomas. Mol Cell Biol 1997;17(8):4782–91.

[92] Yan W, Young AZ, Soares VC, et al. High incidence of T-cell tumors in E2A-null mice and E2A/Id1 double-knockout mice. Mol Cell Biol 1997;17(12):7317–27.

[93] Hertel CB, Zhou XG, Hamilton-Dutoit SJ, et al. Loss of B cell identity correlates with loss of B cell-specific transcription factors in Hodgkin/Reed-Sternberg cells of classical Hodgkin's lymphoma. Oncogene 2002;21(32):4908–20.

[94] Akala OO, Clarke MF. Hematopoietic stem cell self-renewal. Curr Opin Genet Dev 2006;16(5):496–501.

[95] Kato Y, Iwama A, Tadokoro Y, et al. Selective activation of STAT5 unveils its role in stem cell self-renewal in normal and leukemic hematopoiesis. J Exp Med 2005;202(1):169–79.

[96] Orlic D, Anderson S, Biesecker LG, et al. Pluripotent hematopoietic stem cells contain high levels of mRNA for c-kit, GATA-2, p45 NF-E2, and c-myb and low levels or no mRNA for c-fms and the receptors for granulocyte colony-stimulating factor and interleukins 5 and 7. Proc Natl Acad Sci USA 1995;92(10):4601–5.

[97] Tsai FY, Keller G, Kuo FC, et al. An early haematopoietic defect in mice lacking the transcription factor GATA-2. Nature 1994;371(6494):221–6.

[98] Antonchuk J, Sauvageau G, Humphries RK. HOXB4-induced expansion of adult hematopoietic stem cells ex vivo. Cell 2002;109(1):39–45.

[99] Zeng H, Yucel R, Kosan C, et al. Transcription factor Gfi1 regulates self-renewal and engraftment of hematopoietic stem cells. EMBO J 2004;23(20):4116–25.

[100] Park IK, Qian D, Kiel M, et al. Bmi-1 is required for maintenance of adult self-renewing haematopoietic stem cells. Nature 2003;423(6937):302–5.

[101] van der Lugt NM, Alkema M, Berns A, et al. The Polycomb-group homolog Bmi-1 is a regulator of murine Hox gene expression. Mech Dev 1996;58(1–2):153–64.

[102] Duncan AW, Rattis FM, DiMascio LN, et al. Integration of Notch and Wnt signaling in hematopoietic stem cell maintenance. Nat Immunol 2005;6(3):314–22.

[103] Reya T, Duncan AW, Ailles L, et al. A role for Wnt signalling in self-renewal of haematopoietic stem cells. Nature 2003;423(6938):409–14.

[104] Schneider EM, Torlakovic E, Stuhler A, et al. The early transcription factor GATA-2 is expressed in classical Hodgkin's lymphoma. J Pathol 2004;204(5):538–45.

[105] Kapp U, Yeh WC, Patterson B, et al. Interleukin 13 is secreted by and stimulates the growth of Hodgkin and Reed-Sternberg cells. J Exp Med 1999;189(12):1939–46.

[106] Kumano K, Chiba S, Shimizu K, et al. Notch1 inhibits differentiation of hematopoietic cells by sustaining GATA-2 expression. Blood 2001;98(12):3283–9.

[107] Dukers DF, van Galen JC, Giroth C, et al. Unique polycomb gene expression pattern in Hodgkin's lymphoma and Hodgkin's lymphoma-derived cell lines. Am J Pathol 2004; 164(3):873–81.

[108] Raaphorst FM, van Kemenade FJ, Blokzijl T, et al. Coexpression of BMI-1 and EZH2 polycomb group genes in Reed-Sternberg cells of Hodgkin's disease. Am J Pathol 2000;157(3):709–15.

[109] Nagel S, Burek C, Venturini L, et al. Comprehensive analysis of homeobox genes in Hodgkin's lymphoma cell lines identifies dysregulated expression of HOXB9 mediated via ERK5 signaling and BMI1. Blood 2007;109(7):3015–23.

The Potential Role of Innate Immunity in the Pathogenesis of Hodgkin's Lymphoma

Gunilla Enblad, MD, PhD[a],*, Daniel Molin, MD, PhD[a],
Ingrid Glimelius, MD[a], Marie Fischer, PhD[a,b],
Gunnar Nilsson, PhD[b]

[a]Department of Oncology, Radiology, and Clinical Immunology, Section of Oncology,
Uppsala University Hospital, Rudbeck Laboratory C11, S-751 85 Uppsala, Sweden
[b]Clinical Immunology and Allergy, Department of Medicine, Karolinska Institutet, KS L2:04,
17176 Stockholm, Sweden

Malignancies are composed of several cell types besides the mutated tumor cells. These make up the microenvironment that was proved to be important for tumor development. The microenvironment can consist of fibroblasts, epithelial cells, endothelial cells, and cells of the innate and adaptive immune system [1]. Although activation of adaptive immune cells in response to the tumor might lead to eradication of the tumor cells, chronic activation of innate immune cells might promote tumorigenesis [2]. Innate immune cells, such as dendritic cells, macrophages, mast cells, neutrophils, basophils, and eosinophils, are the first line of defense against pathogens and other danger signals. In particular, dendritic cells, macrophages, and mast cells act as sentinel cells in the tissue and can respond rapidly to signs of distress. Cells of the innate immune system have the capacity to release a myriad of mediators, such as cytokines, chemokines, growth factors, eicosanoids, histamine, matrix remodeling proteases, and reactive oxygen species, leading to an inflammatory response. Today, it is evident that mediators released from activated innate immune cells promote tumorigenesis by their effects on cell growth and survival, tissue remodeling, angiogenesis, and suppression of antitumor adaptive immune responses [2,3].

Hodgkin's lymphoma (HL) is a good example of a malignancy in which the tumor microenvironment is of great importance for the development and progression of tumors [4]. HL is characterized by the peculiar microanatomic presentation of the affected lymph nodes with only a few malignant cells (often

*Corresponding author. Department of Oncology, Radiology and Clinical Immunology, Section of Oncology, Uppsala University, S-751 85 Uppsala, Sweden. E-mail address: Gunilla.Enblad@onkologi.uu.se (G. Enblad).

0889-8588/07/$ – see front matter
doi:10.1016/j.hoc.2007.07.007
© 2007 Elsevier Inc. All rights reserved.
hemonc.theclinics.com

less than 1% of cells in the tumor tissue) and an abundance of inflammatory cells. The sparse Hodgkin's and Reed-Sternberg (HRS) cells are surrounded by a reactive infiltrate composed of T and B cells mixed with cells of the innate immune system, (eg, neutrophils, macrophages, eosinophils, and mast cells). A complex network of interactions mediated by cytokines, chemokines, and cell–cell contact exists between the different cell types in this disease and seems vital for its development and progression [5,6]. The dependency of HRS cells on their microenvironment is supported by the difficulty of maintaining these cells in culture, the inability of primary HRS cells to survive in immunodeficient mice, and that HRS cells are rarely found in the peripheral blood [4].

In keeping with traditional tumor research, a substantial effort has been made to investigate the malignant HRS cells, whereas the inflammatory cells have been, until recently, dismissed as blind followers. As a result, the contribution of certain cell types to tumor development has been neglected in the past. The mast cell is an example of this because its presence in HL has been noted but its potential contribution to HL pathology has attracted little attention to date. In this article we present plausible roles of the innate immune cells—neutrophils, eosinophils, macrophages, and mast cells—in the tumor development in HL, based on experimental and clinical data. For example, several of these cells express various tumor necrosis factor (TNF)–like receptors and ligands that are believed to be of importance for HL pathology [5,7,8]. Furthermore, eosinophils and mast cells seem to contribute to a worse prognosis and tissue fibrosis in HL [9–11].

CELLS OF THE INNATE IMMUNITY AND THEIR ROLE IN HODGKIN'S LYMPHOMA
Eosinophils
The eosinophilic granulocyte has long been recognized as an important cell in asthma and allergy. It is also known for its physiologic functions in the defense against various pathogens and in wound healing. Most of its functions are mediated by different proteins released from its cytoplasmic granules [12]. Lately, the importance of those cells in relation to tumors has also been demonstrated, mostly in cancers where they seem to have a protective effect. In HL, however, they seem to play another role, as is described later.

Basic biology
The eosinophilic granulocyte is morphologically characterized by a bilobular nucleus and cytoplasmic granules, stained by eosin. They are derived from $CD34^+$ hematopoietic progenitor cells and mature in the bone marrow. Eosinophils are found circulating in peripheral blood and can remain in the tissue for days or even weeks. Physiologically, the eosinophils are active in the body's defense against parasites and viruses. They also initiate inflammatory processes and modulate innate and adaptive immunity [12]. Other possible roles for these cells are in wound healing and in the defense against carcinomas, either by way

of their cytotoxic granule proteins or by interaction with other cells in the immune system [13,14].

The cytoplasmic granules of the eosinophil contain several basic proteins: major basic protein, eosinophil protein X or eosinophil-derived neurotoxin [15], eosinophil peroxidase, and eosinophil cationic protein (ECP). There are also other proteins present in the granules, such as IL-2, IL-4, IL-5, catalase, IL-6 [16], IL-10, IL-12, IL-13, IL-16, IL-18, transforming growth factor (TGF)α, TGFβ, TNF-α [17,18], and bacterial permeability increasing protein. Triggering of eosinophils also lead to secretion of chemokines, such as RANTES (CCL5) and eotaxin (CCL11) [12].

Diseases other than HL that are intimately associated with eosinophils include asthma, allergy, atopic dermatitis, and hypereosinophilic syndrome. Suggested roles for the eosinophils in these conditions are, for example, tissue destruction and remodeling [19].

One protein that seems to be of particular interest is the ECP, described in Uppsala in 1977 [20]. The protein is a single-chain peptide of 133 amino acids, with a molecular weight ranging from 18 to 22 kDa, depending on the level of glycosylation [21]. ECP is a ribonuclease [12] and member of the RNase A superfamily [13]. ECP has a capacity for parasite killing, which is probably one of its main physiologic functions. Furthermore, it has antibacterial and also antiviral functions. ECP also affects human cells (eg, fibroblast function) because it inhibits proteoglycan degradation [22]. This mechanism can stimulate fibrosis. ECP also affects coagulation [23], plasma cells, and B cells, inhibiting Ig production by these cells [24,25].

Distribution in Hodgkin's lymphoma
HL has been associated with eosinophilia in the blood, bone marrow, and tumor tissue. In the tumor tissue, many cases of HL show heavy eosinophilia [10,26]. Eosinophils are distributed relatively evenly in cellular areas of the tumors but can also be found in sheets with a high concentration of eosinophils. A few of these eosinophils are situated in close proximity to the HRS cells (Fig. 1).

The number of eosinophils has been reported to vary between histopathologic subtypes. A correlation between abundant eosinophils and nodular sclerosis (NS) HL histology has been described in some materials [10,27] but not all [11]. Unpublished data from our own more recent investigations confirms that there is no correlation to NSHL histology (Ingrid Glimelius, MD, unpublished data, 2006). There seem to be no cases with prominent eosinophilia in nodular lymphocytic predominance HL [11].

Correlation to prognosis
A relationship has been shown between HL cases with abundant eosinophils in the tumor and poor prognosis [10], and whereas this has been confirmed in a larger study [11] it was also questioned in a smaller study [27]. The correlation to survival is especially pronounced in NSHL histology. Bone marrow eosinophilia in patients who have HL does not affect prognosis [28], whereas blood eosinophilia in HL is associated with a favorable prognosis [29].

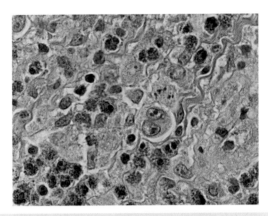

Fig. 1. Hodgkin's lymphoma tissue stained with hematoxylin-eosin, original magnification ×1000, showing a Reed-Sternberg cell surrounded by numerous eosinophils (in pink).

In other malignant tumors, such as colon cancer [30] and head and neck cancer [31], presence of tumor-associated eosinophilia is associated with a comparatively good prognosis. These data suggest a special role of eosinophils in HL tumors.

The better prognosis in tumors other than HL is assumed to be attributable to the cytotoxic activity of the eosinophils [31]. Interestingly, in historical materials, prognosis in patients who have NS histology in general is relatively good, but patients who have NS histology and eosinophilia in the tumors have a poor prognosis [10,11].

Possible interactions in Hodgkin's lymphoma

The exact mechanisms behind the presence of numerous eosinophils in HL tumors is as yet unclear but could be because of secretion of IL-5 [32], IL-9 [33], CCL28, and granulocyte-macrophage colony stimulating factor (GM-CSF) [34] by the HRS cells, or eotaxin (CCL11) secreted from fibroblasts and macrophages, which are stimulated by TNF-α from the HRS cells [35]. The eosinophils could also affect the mast cells, because histamine release from mast cells is stimulated by ECP [36].

The poorer prognosis in eosinophil-rich cases has in one study been proposed to be because of the expression of a ligand to the CD30 receptor (CD30 L/CD153), a member of the TNF/nerve growth factor (NGF) superfamily. This interaction can stimulate HRS cell proliferation [37].

Of particular interest in HL and the peculiar accumulation of fibrosis in NSHL is the eosinophils' production of TGFβ and subsequent stimulation of fibroblasts [38]. TGFβ levels in urine are elevated in NSHL patients [39], and much of this TGFβ is secreted from eosinophils [38]. Another possible mechanism for this is the ability of ECP to inhibit proteoglycan degradation in fibroblasts. ECP can also stimulate fibroblasts [22], which could contribute to the NSHL histology by creating fibrotic bands if high levels of ECP are present in HL.

High levels of serum-eosinophil cationic protein (S-ECP) are present in many cases of HL and correlate to the number of eosinophils in the tumors. S-ECP correlates to high erythrocyte sedimentation rate, suggesting a relation to inflammation, and also NSHL histology, advanced-stage disease, and bulky disease [40]. Furthermore, a single nucleotide polymorphism (434[G>C]) in the ECP gene, previously shown to correlate to allergy, might affect the level of inflammation in HL (Daniel Molin, MD, PhD, unpublished data, 2002).

Neutrophils

Basic biology

Neutrophil polymorphonuclear leukocytes are derived from hematopoietic stem cells in the bone marrow and are the most abundant type of white blood cell. The neutrophils are the first line of defense against infectious agents, are rapidly recruited to sites of injury or infection, and can act as phagocytes. The neutrophils have a multilobulated nucleus and the cytoplasm is filled with granules. The granules are of three types: specific, azurophilic, and tertiary granules. They release their enzyme content on stimulation. Neutrophils are regulated by cytokines, including hematopoietic growth factors. They also release small amounts of some cytokines, including IL-1, IL-6, TNFα, and GM-CSF.

Distribution in Hodgkin's lymphoma

Neutrophils are found in the tumor tissue and distributed among other infiltrating cells. Often the number of neutrophils is lower than the number of eosinophils. The role of neutrophils has not as yet been thoroughly studied. It has long been noted, however, that there is an increase in neutrophil number in the blood of patients who have HL and many patients have slight to moderate leukocytosis.

Correlation to prognosis

An increase in leukocyte counts is correlated to a poor prognosis and a leukocyte level greater than $15 \times 10^9/L$ is an adverse prognostic factor according to the International Prognostic score [41].

Possible interactions in Hodgkin's lymphoma

There are many cytokines produced by the HRS cells that might contribute to the accumulation of neutrophils (eg, G-CSF, GM-CSF, TGF-β, and IL-8). IL-8 has also been shown to be produced by mast cells on activation of CD30 L by way of CD30 [42]. Leukocytosis in HL has been correlated to high levels of IL-10 in one study [43] but not in others [44,45].

Mast Cells

Mast cells are recognized key effector cells during allergic reactions and as such they have long been the main interest for allergologists. Time has proved mast cells to be multifunctional cells that are not only important in IgE-mediated immune responses but also as regulatory cells in innate and acquired immunity. Furthermore, they have been implicated in various physiologic and pathologic conditions [46]. Their functional diversity is attributable to the release of selected mediators from a myriad of proinflammatory and immuno-regulatory molecules in response to various stimuli. One of the most interesting advances in recent mast cell biology research is the observation that mast cells participate in tumorigenesis [47,48].

Basic biology
Mast cells were named by the German scientist Paul Erlich, who in his thesis in 1878 described a connective tissue cell with a characteristic basophilic staining pattern. One of the early findings of Ehrlich and his student Westphal was the accumulation of mast cells in tumor tissues. During the following hundred years many publications have described the presence of mast cells in several different malignancies, but their role in tumorigenesis is still not clear [48].

Mast cells are derived from pluripotent $CD34^+$ hematopoietic stem cells within the bone marrow, but unlike other leukocytes they do not mature at that site. Rather, immature $CD34^+c\text{-}Kit^+CD13^+$ progenitors circulate in the blood and are recruited into vascularized tissues where they undergo final differentiation under the influence of microenvironmental factors [49,50]. The main regulator of mast cell extravasation, proliferation, and differentiation is stem cell factor (SCF), the ligand for the c-kit tyrosine kinase receptor consti-tutively expressed on the mast cell surface. Although SCF is by far the most important promoter of mast cell development, many other factors, such as IL-3, IL-4, IL-5, IL-6, IL-9, nerve growth factor (NGF), chemokines, and retinoids, contribute to mast cell differentiation either synergistically or antag-onistically in a complex network. During the maturation process mast cells ac-quire their typical granulated morphology and begin to express the high-affinity receptor for IgE (FcεRI), which is one of the classic markers for these cells.

The tissue microenvironment has a profound impact on the development and subsequent phenotypic expression of mast cells. Depending on differences in the cytokine milieu and cell interactions occurring in various tissues, mast cells develop heterogeneous phenotypes and functional characteristics. Even so, two major categories can be distinguished. One population contains the proteases tryptase and chymase in the granules and is thus designated MC_{TC}, whereas the remaining population stores only tryptase and is abbrevi-ated accordingly as MC_T [51]. In tissue localization, MC_{TC} predominates in the skin and intestinal submucosa, whereas MC_T is the predominant subtype in the lung and intestinal lamina propria.

Characteristic features of mast cells are the abundance of electron-dense granules and the capacity to release a great variety of inflammatory mediators. On activation, mast cells have the ability to release mediators in three different ways. Depending on the stimuli all three or just one or two of them can be engaged. The most rapid response is degranulation, which happens within 15 minutes after activation, because of aggregation of the high-affinity IgE receptor. During degranulation, histamine, proteases, heparin, and preformed cytokines are released. Mast cells also synthesize and secrete various eicosanoids; leukotriene C4 and prostaglandin D2 being the most prominent. This secretion takes place within 30 minutes after activation. Finally, mast cells have the capacity to synthesize many different cytokines, chemokines, and growth factors that are released hours after activation. The spectrum of cytokines/chemokines/growth factors that are released depends on the mast cell phenotype, environment, and the trigger that induces the de novo protein synthesis.

It is thus clear that mast cell activation can have various consequences depending on what is released from the activated cells. Mast cell mediators can cause vascular effects (histamine, PGD2, LTC4, VEGF); stimulation of angiogenesis (IL-8, proteases, VEGF); tissue remodeling, such as fibrosis (proteases, TGFβ); cell recruitment (chemokines, TNF-α, PGD2, LTB4); immunomodulation (IL-4, IL-13, CD40 L/CD154, CD30 L/CD153); and stimulation of granulocytes (GM-CSF, IL-3, IL-5).

Mast cells in tumors

An association between mast cells and tumors is clear, but the relevance of this relationship is not. There is a growing body of data indicating that mast cells promote tumor growth and metastasis by the release of various mediators rather than by providing active defense against tumors (reviewed in [47]). Direct evidence for the contribution of mast cell–derived proteases during experimental skin carcinogenesis in mice has been reported [52]. Mast cells can stimulate tumor growth either directly through cell–cell interactions and release of cytokines and growth factors, or indirectly by facilitating angiogenesis and tissue remodeling. Neovascularization is a critical step for tumor development to prevent hypoxia. Mast cells are associated with angiogenesis in tumors, such as hemangioma, carcinomas, lymphoma, and multiple myeloma [53], but not in HL [54]. Many mediators produced by mast cells are known to promote angiogenesis either directly, such as histamine, IL-8, and VEGF, or indirectly by proteases that degrade extracellular matrix leading to the release of matrix-associated growth factors. A potential role for mast cells in tumor development is thus evident, but to fully understand their role in the process, the mechanisms behind the accumulation of these cells in tumor areas and the specific triggers that set them into action need to be defined.

Distribution of mast cells in tumors

There are several reports on the presence of mast cells in HL-affected lymph nodes [8,55,56]. Most HL cases (>90%) and all histopathologic subtypes show mast cell infiltration [8]. The numbers of mast cells vary slightly between histopathologic subtypes. The highest numbers are seen in the NSHL subtype (approximately 12 mast cells/high-power field [HPF]) [8]. Increased numbers of eosinophils are also associated with NSHL, and mixed cellularity HL also has many eosinophils [10,11]. This finding is interesting considering that cross-talk between mast cells, eosinophils, and fibroblasts can contribute to the development of fibrosis [57]. Fewer mast cells are found in LD and LPn subtypes (5.5 and 7.5 mast cells/HPF, respectively) [8,55].

Mast cells are distributed mainly in the sinuses and the interfollicular areas, and not as much in the zones [56]. In NSHL they are frequently found in areas of fibrosis (Fig. 2). Occasionally they can be found in close contact with HRS cells.

Correlation to prognosis
If mast cells are a part of the cancer development in HL one would anticipate that mast cell numbers in HL correlate to negative prognostic factors (Table 1). Indeed, increased mast cell number in HL correlates to high white blood cell counts (WBC) and low blood hemoglobin. Mast cell infiltration into affected lymph nodes also correlates with worse disease-free survival [9] (Fig. 3).

Possible interactions between mast cells and Hodgkin's and Reed-Sternberg cells in Hodgkin's lymphoma
Given that mast cells increase in number and correlate to poorer prognosis in HL, the question remains as to how these cells contribute to the tumorigenesis in HL. We here discuss how mast cells can be recruited to the lymph node and how mast cells and HRS cells can interact with each other.

Mast cell migration can be induced by various chemoattractants, of which the chemokines are an important part. HL is a tumor with disturbed cytokine features, whereby the aberrant cytokine production contributes not only to proliferation of HRS cells but also to the maintenance of an appropriate environment for the tumor cells [6]. Among the cytokines produced are several chemokines that contribute to the composition of the inflammatory infiltrate in HL [58]. CCL5/RANTES is one of these chemokines and is produced by HRS cells and possibly by other cells in the tumor [59–61]. Mast cells express two receptors, CCR1 and CCR4, that can bind CCL5 and thereby induce mast cell migration [62,63]. CCL5 thus plays a plausible role in the accumulation of mast cells in HL [61].

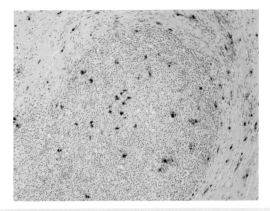

Fig. 2. Hodgkin's lymphoma tissue immunohistochemically stained with the monoclonal antibody G3, recognizing the mast cell–specific protein tryptase, original magnification ×100; numerous mast cells are seen in fibrotic and in cellular areas.

Table 1
Relationship between eosinophils, mast cells, and clinical and tumor biologic characteristics

	High eosinophil infiltration	High mast cell infiltration
Mean cell no. (range) in HL-affected lymph nodes	123 (0–1451)/10 HPF[a]	19 (0–101)/10 HPF
Mean cell no. (range) from 10 reactive lymph nodes	2 (0–8)/10 HPF[a]	23 (0–86)/10 HPF[a]
Negative prognostic factor	Yes	Yes
Correlation to high ESR	Yes	Yes
Correlation to NS histology	No	Yes
Age	Younger patients have more eosinophils, $P = .03$[a]	No correlation[a]
Correlation to IL-9 positive HRS	Yes	Yes
Correlation to high microvessel count	No	No

[a]Ingrid Glimelius, MD, unpublished data, 2006.

Within the tumor tissue mast cells can interact with HRS cells and other cells and thus contribute to the tumor progression (Fig. 4). One important pathway is the CD30–CD30 L/CD153 interaction between HRS cells and inflammatory cells that constitute a bidirectional interaction between the cells. CD30 was originally identified as an HL-associated antigen highly expressed on HRS cells [64]. The CD30 molecule belongs to the TNF receptor superfamily (TNFR), along with, for example, CD40 and FAS, and is a type I transmembrane glycosylated protein with an extracellular N-terminal domain [65,66]. The

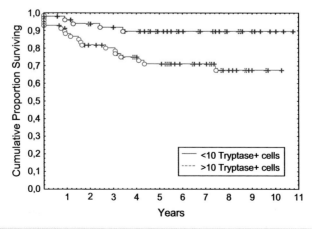

Fig. 3. Progression-free survival in patients who have few and many mast cells.

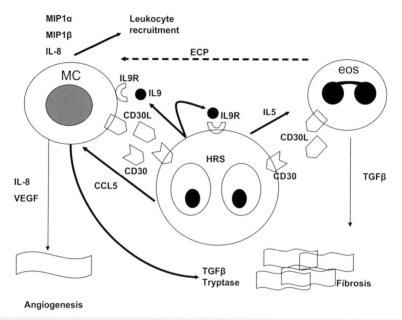

Fig. 4. Possible interactions between HRS cells, mast cells, and eosinophils.

ubiquitous expression on HRS cells in almost every case of HL makes CD30 a useful marker for this malignancy and suggests an important role for this molecule in tumor development in HL. The CD30 ligand (CD153) is expressed on several cell types, including eosinophils, neutrophils, and mast cells [8,37,67]. The extracellular part can be proteolytically cleaved by a zinc metalloproteinase to produce a soluble form of CD30 (sCD30) that can be measured in cell culture supernatants and serum samples [68,69]. In healthy patients sCD30 is generally absent or is present at very low levels, whereas elevated levels correlate with negative prognostic factors in HL, such as advanced stage, high tumor burden, and B symptoms (ie, weight loss, night sweats, fever) [70]. It is therefore suggested that levels of sCD30 can be used as a prognostic factor [71].

It is of particular interest that mast cells constitute most (66%) of the CD30 L–positive cells in HL [8]. The relevance of CD30 activation in HL pathology is still uncertain and only a limited number of studies have addressed the contribution of CD30 L–expressing cells. The activation of HRS cells by CD30 L results in a proliferative response in the tumor cells, and this has been speculated to be one reason for the negative prognostic impact associated with the presence of large numbers of eosinophils and mast cells in HL [7,9,37,72].

Interaction between CD30 and its ligand constitutes a bidirectional interaction, whereby not only CD30-positive cells can be activated by CD30 L but also the CD30 L–positive cell can be activated by CD30. The finding that the CD30 L molecule is capable of so-called "reverse signaling" shed yet more light on the possible role of CD30 L–expressing cells in HL. Activation of neutrophils or mast cells with CD30 causes secretion of IL-8 [42,73]. CD30 activation of mast cells constitutes a unique mechanism of cell activation/triggering because they do not degranulate or release leukotrienes, but secrete only a specific set of chemokines, including IL-8, MIP-1a, and MIP-1b [42]. These chemokines are involved in the recruitment of granulocytes, lymphocytes, and monocytes, cells commonly found in HL. Through this bidirectional interaction mast cells thus have dual roles by stimulating the growth of tumor cells and by contributing to the recruitment of inflammatory cells to the tumor.

Antigen-Presenting Cells: Macrophages and Dendritic Cells

Basic biology

Macrophages are derived from hematopoietic stem cells and differentiated from monocytes, which are mobile phagocytic cells. Macrophages are widely distributed in almost all tissue types, such as Langerhans cells in the skin and Kupffer cells in the liver. Macrophages are heterogeneous and involved in all stages of the immune response. One important role of macrophages in the immune system is to digest pathogens and present antigens together with the MHC class II antigen, thereby stimulating the adaptive immune response. Macrophages are regulated by various cytokines and are also stimulated by histamine released from mast cells.

Dendritic cells (DCs) are immune cells whose main function is to process and present antigen. There are four types of DCs: lymphoid DCs, DC cells, plasmacytoid DCs, and follicular DCs. The DCs are probably of hematopoietic linage although the origin of follicular DCs is disputed. DCs circulate in the blood as immature precursors before migration into peripheral tissues. Within tissues DCs differentiate and become active in taking up and processing antigens. DCs are a major source of cytokines and have been shown to produce IL-1, IL-6, IL-7, IL-10, IL-12, and IL-15. They also express CD40 and are stimulated by CD40 L/CD154 and are important for the germinal center function in the lymph nodes [92].

Distribution in Hodgkin's lymphoma

Macrophages have mainly been studied in HL as a possible cell of origin for the HRS cells. Following the evidence that HRS cells are derived from lymphoid cells the studies have focused on chemokines derived from or related to monocytes/macrophages. HRS cells have been shown to express the macrophage-related chemokine MDC, mainly in NS [93].

Recently, Sánchez-Aguilera and colleagues [94] presented a study in which they have studied whole tumor tissue in 29 HL samples using microarray technology. They found two clusters of genes related to host tumor response and tumor microenvironment. One signature that was related to a group with unfavorable prognosis included overexpression of genes expressed by specific subpopulations of T cells, macrophages (STAT1, ALDH1A1, and LYZ), and plasmacytoid dendritic cells (ITM2A). In a validation set they performed immunohistochemistry on tissue microarray from 235 patients and showed that high expression of STAT1 and ALDH1A1 was related to a poor prognosis. The expression of STAT1 was predominately in macrophages.

Correlation to prognosis
The correlation to prognosis has not been studied other than the above-mentioned study.

Possible interactions in Hodgkin's lymphoma
Macrophages and DCs are key players in the innate immune system and because they express and are stimulated by several cytokines, numerous interactions with HRS cells and the bystander cells in the HL tissue are possible. Although these interactions have not been studied in any detail, serum levels of IL-10 have been shown to be of importance in HL [44] and most probably the CD40-CD40 ligand interactions also [92].

EXPRESSION AND FUNCTION OF IL-9 IN HODGKIN'S LYMPHOMA

HL has an abnormal production of cytokines, and the presence of reactive cells in HL tissue is probably because of the production of specific cytokines and chemokines by HRS cells [74,75]. One example of such a cytokine is IL-9, which is produced by and acts on HRS cells and inflammatory cells [33,76].

IL-9 is a multifunctional cytokine that in addition to its activities in immune and inflammatory responses, such as asthma [77], has a suggested role in promoting oncogenesis [78]. In malignant tumors IL-9 is almost exclusively related to HL and anaplastic large cell lymphomas [76]. The main source of IL-9 is activated Th2 lymphocytes, but other cell types, including mast cells, can also produce IL-9 [78]. The HL cell lines HDLM2 and KMH2 express IL-9 and respond to IL-9 stimulation. Based on this observation an autocrine loop has been postulated, in which IL-9 is active as a growth factor for the HRS cells [79]. IL-9 also is synergistic with SCF to promote the growth of cultured HRS cells of the KMH2 cell line [80].

In tumor biopsies, IL-9 expression is present in the cytoplasm of HRS cells in about 50% of the cases and expression of interleukin-9 receptor (IL-9R) is seen in about 20% [33]. An increased serum level of IL-9 is found in about 40% of the patients who have HL [81]. A correlation between serum levels and expression in the tumors indicates that the HRS cells are the source of the IL-9 in serum [81].

Because of the multifunctional role of IL-9, acting on mast cells and eosinophils [82–84], it is reasonable to believe that IL-9 is of importance for the surrounding innate cells in HL. IL-9 expression by HRS cells correlates to the number of eosinophils and mast cells in HL tumors [33]. It can therefore be hypothesized that IL-9, in addition to other cytokines produced by HRS cells, has a stimulatory effect on these cells in the tumors. That IL-9R expression has been observed on cells resembling mast cells in HL also supports this hypothesis [33].

Despite a clear correlation between IL-9 and the number of eosinophils and mast cells, both of which have prognostic importance in HL [9,10], and the possible autocrine stimulation of the HRS cells, any influence of IL-9 on survival in HL has not been detected [33]. Patients with IL-9 positive HL tumors have higher WBC and erythrocyte sedimentation rate (ESR), however, both of which are parameters related to inflammation and poor prognosis [33]. High levels of IL-9 in serum also correlate to negative prognostic factors, such as high ESR, high WBC, B symptoms, and advanced stage [81].

From a tumor biology point of view it is also of interest that IL-9 expression in the tumors and in sera correlates to NS histology. This correlation indicates that IL-9 and its receptor, among other cytokines, are also involved in fibroblast activation, leading to the dense fibrosis seen in these tumors [33,81,85].

INNATE CELLS AND ANGIOGENESIS IN HODGKIN'S LYMPHOMA

Angiogenesis, the formation and stabilization of new vessels from pre-existing blood vessels, has a well-established role in the development of tumors [86]. So far, the information about angiogenesis and its possible mechanisms in patients who have HL is limited.

High microvessel density (MVD) or high microvessel count (MVC) predicts poor prognosis in HL, shown in two recent reports [54,87], and MVD increased with disease progression in 7 out of 11 cases of classical HL [88]. VEGF, a major angiogenic molecule, is expressed by HRS in about 70% of HL lymph nodes; however, only a weak correlation between VEGF expression of the HRS cells and MVD is shown [89]. Also the HL cell lines L425 and KM-H2 express VEGF [89].

The mechanism behind angiogenesis is probably a complex interplay between the malignant cells and the surrounding tissue, and in particular the innate cells. Mast cells are associated with angiogenesis in solid tumors and in hematologic malignancies, such as B-cell non-Hodgkin's lymphoma and multiple myeloma [53]. Mast cells express several factors that can affect angiogenesis directly and indirectly, including VEGF, basic fibroblast growth factor, TGFβ, TNFα, IL-8, histamine, tryptase, matrix metalloproteinase-9, and heparin [90]. No correlation between high mast cell count and MVC in HL was observed in one study, however [54]. This lack of correlation might indicate different pathways for the proliferation of microvessels in HL compared with other lymphomas. A contribution of mast cells to microvessel stimulation cannot be ruled out, although this is not reflected in mast cell numbers, because mast cells express several angiogenic factors and show large variations in the production of these. Reactive macrophages in HL were positive for VEGF, indicating that they may contribute to angiogenesis in HL [89].

The knowledge about possible contribution of other innate cells, such as eosinophils, neutrophils, and monocytes, to angiogenesis in HL is still limited. Because most leukocytes produce numerous angiogenic factors it is likely that these cells can also contribute to the formation of new blood vessels in HL [91]. These cells also generate angiogenesis inhibitors, however, so their overall role in initiating or terminating angiogenesis depends on the temporal and spatial balance of these molecules [91]. This has to be evaluated for each cell type, each factor, and each disease separately.

IS THERE ANY CORRELATION BETWEEN ALLERGY AND HODGKIN'S LYMPHOMA?

Because cells of the innate immune system have been observed in HL an association between HL and allergy has been suspected. Earlier studies have focused on increased levels of IgE found in patients who have HL and an association between elevated IgE levels and NS histology and B symptoms. The hypothesis has been that elevated IgE levels are polyclonal and reflect a suppressor T-cell dysfunction. Several studies have addressed the hypothesis that people who have allergic conditions (eg, asthma or hay fever) have a reduced risk for various malignancies. The idea is that allergy is a hyperreactive state of the immune system leading to enhanced immune surveillance and a decreased proliferation of aberrant cells. None of the studies have had enough patients to calculate the HL risk. Grulich and colleagues [95] found that atopic conditions were associated with a reduced risk for non-Hodgkin's lymphoma. The effect was most prominent in people who had early birth order and, as a consequence of that, a Th2-dominated immune response. Other studies have not been able to confirm these results, however [96]. There is, to our knowledge, only one study specifically addressing the prognosis in patients who have HL with and without atopy. In 1983, Amlot and colleagues [97] published a study showing that patients who had a personal history of atopy had a better prognosis.

NEW THERAPEUTIC STRATEGIES TARGETING INNATE IMMUNE CELLS IN HODGKIN'S LYMPHOMA

HL is an example of a tumor that seems to depend almost totally on the surrounding microenvironment of cells of the innate and adaptive immune system. It is tempting to speculate that future treatments could target these immune cells, thus leaving the HRS cells without their required support and consequently doomed to apoptosis. The dependence of immune cells is probably different among patients. If the pathways could be delineated for every individual patient, or group of patients, targeted therapy may then be possible. Antibodies directed toward IL5 exist and have been studied in the treatment of asthma [98]. Because of lack of effect the antibodies have never reached the market. Those antibodies could be of interest to try in eosinophil-dependent HL (if such an entity exists). Another possibility is to take advantage of new knowledge in the field of allergology, especially the idea of inducing apoptosis of mast cells. IL-9 could also be a potential target because of its high expression in many patients who have HL. Finally, the innate immune cells could be involved in the angiogenesis of HL, although we were not able to show a correlation between MVD and prognosis. New drugs directed toward tumor angiogenesis could also be of importance for patients who have HL.

SUMMARY

HL is a peculiar disease containing few tumor cells surrounded by an infiltrate of innate and adaptive cells of the immune system. Numerous studies have shown that the HRS cells are active cytokine producers and they probably attract the immune cells by this cytokine secretion. In this article we have described some known interactions between HRS cells and cells of the innate immune system that clearly contribute to the pathogenesis of the disease along with the prognosis. Our hypothesis is that different immune cells or varying proportions of immune cells are important in different patients (ie, mast cell–driven, eosinophil-driven, or macrophage-driven HL). If these pathways can be further clarified, specific treatment can be introduced.

Acknowledgments
GE and GN are supported by The Swedish Cancer Foundation.

References
[1] Hanahan D, Weinberg RA. The hallmarks of cancer. Cell 2000;100(1):57–70.
[2] de Visser KE, Eichten A, Coussens LM. Paradoxical roles of the immune system during cancer development. Nat Rev Cancer 2006;6(1):24–37.
[3] Balkwill F, Mantovani A. Inflammation and cancer: back to Virchow? Lancet 2001; 357(9255):539–45.
[4] Kuppers R, Hansmann ML. The Hodgkin's and Reed/Sternberg cell. Int J Biochem Cell Biol 2005;37(3):511–7.
[5] Pinto A, Gattei V, Zagonel V, et al. Hodgkin's disease: a disorder of dysregulated cellular cross-talk. Biotherapy 1998;10(4):309–20.
[6] Gruss HJ, Pinto A, Duyster J, et al. Hodgkin's disease: a tumor with disturbed immunological pathways. Immunol Today 1997;18(4):156–63.
[7] Pinto A, Aldinucci D, Gloghini A, et al. The role of eosinophils in the pathobiology of Hodgkin's disease. Ann Oncol 1997;8(Suppl 2):89–96.
[8] Molin D, Fischer M, Xiang Z, et al. Mast cells express functional CD30 ligand and are the predominant CD30L-positive cells in Hodgkin's disease. Br J Haematol 2001;114(3):616–23.
[9] Molin D, Edstrom A, Glimelius I, et al. Mast cell infiltration correlates with poor prognosis in Hodgkin's lymphoma. Br J Haematol 2002;119(1):122–4.
[10] Enblad G, Sundstrom C, Glimelius B. Infiltration of eosinophils in Hodgkin's disease involved lymph nodes predicts prognosis. Hematol Oncol 1993;11(4):187–93.
[11] von Wasielewski R, Seth S, Franklin J, et al. Tissue eosinophilia correlates strongly with poor prognosis in nodular sclerosing Hodgkin's disease, allowing for known prognostic factors. Blood 2000;95(4):1207–13.
[12] Rothenberg ME, Hogan SP. The eosinophil. Annu Rev Immunol 2006;24:147–74.
[13] Venge P, Bystrom J, Carlson M, et al. Eosinophil cationic protein (ECP): molecular and biological properties and the use of ECP as a marker of eosinophil activation in disease. Clin Exp Allergy 1999;29(9):1172–86.

[14] Trulson A, Nilsson S, Venge P. The eosinophil granule proteins in serum, but not the oxidative metabolism of the blood eosinophils, are increased in cancer. Br J Haematol 1997;98(2): 312–4.

[15] Peterson CG, Venge P. Purification and characterization of a new cationic protein–eosinophil protein-X (EPX)–from granules of human eosinophils. Immunology 1983;50(1): 19–26.

[16] Hamid Q, Barkans J, Meng Q, et al. Human eosinophils synthesize and secrete interleukin-6, in vitro. Blood 1992;80(6):1496–501.

[17] Beil WJ, Weller PF, Tzizik DM, et al. Ultrastructural immunogold localization of tumor necrosis factor-alpha to the matrix compartment of eosinophil secondary granules in patients with idiopathic hypereosinophilic syndrome. J Histochem Cytochem 1993;41(11): 1611–5.

[18] Calafat J, Janssen H, Tool A, et al. The bactericidal/permeability-increasing protein (BPI) is present in specific granules of human eosinophils. Blood 1998;91(12):4770–5.

[19] Levi-Schaffer F, Weg VB. Mast cells, eosinophils and fibrosis. Clin Exp Allergy 1997;27(Suppl 1):64–70.

[20] Olsson I, Venge P, Spitznagel JK, et al. Arginine-rich cationic proteins of human eosinophil granules: comparison of the constituents of eosinophilic and neutrophilic leukocytes. Lab Invest 1977;36(5):493–500.

[21] Peterson CG, Jornvall H, Venge P. Purification and characterization of eosinophil cationic protein from normal human eosinophils. Eur J Haematol 1988;40(5):415–23.

[22] Hernnas J, Sarnstrand B, Lindroth P, et al. Eosinophil cationic protein alters proteoglycan metabolism in human lung fibroblast cultures. Eur J Cell Biol 1992;59(2):352–63.

[23] Venge P, Dahl R, Hallgren R. Enhancement of factor XII dependent reactions by eosinophil cationic protein. Thromb Res 1979;14(4–5):641–9.

[24] Kimata H, Yoshida A, Ishioka C, et al. Inhibition of ongoing immunoglobulin production by eosinophil cationic protein. Clin Immunol Immunopathol 1992;64(1):84–8.

[25] Kimata H, Yoshida A, Ishioka C, et al. Eosinophil cationic protein inhibits immunoglobulin production and proliferation in vitro in human plasma cells. Cell Immunol 1992;141(2): 422–32.

[26] Toth J, Dworak O, Sugar J. Eosinophil predominance in Hodgkin's disease. Z Krebsforsch Klin Onkol Cancer Res Clin Oncol 1977;89(1):107–11.

[27] Axdorph U, Porwit-MacDonald A, Grimfors G, et al. Tissue eosinophilia in relation to immunopathological and clinical characteristics in Hodgkin's disease. Leuk Lymphoma 2001;42(5):1055–65.

[28] Macintyre EA, Vaughan Hudson B, Vaughan Hudson G, et al. Incidence and clinical importance of bone marrow eosinophilia in Hodgkin's disease (BNLI Report No 29). British National Lymphoma Investigation. J Clin Pathol 1987;40(3):245–6.

[29] Vaughan Hudson B, Linch DC, Macintyre EA, et al. Selective peripheral blood eosinophilia associated with survival advantage in Hodgkin's disease (BNLI Report No 31). British National Lymphoma Investigation. J Clin Pathol 1987;40(3):247–50.

[30] Pretlow TP, Keith EF, Cryar AK, et al. Eosinophil infiltration of human colonic carcinomas as a prognostic indicator. Cancer Res 1983;43(6):2997–3000.

[31] Goldsmith MM, Belchis DA, Cresson DH, et al. The importance of the eosinophil in head and neck cancer. Otolaryngol Head Neck Surg 1992;106(1):27–33.

[32] Samoszuk M, Nansen L. Detection of interleukin-5 messenger RNA in Reed-Sternberg cells of Hodgkin's disease with eosinophilia. Blood 1990;75(1):13–6.

[33] Glimelius I, Edstrom A, Amini RM, et al. IL-9 expression contributes to the cellular composition in Hodgkin's lymphoma. Eur J Haematol 2006;76(4):278–83.

[34] Endo M UK, Kitazume K, Iwabe K, et al. Hypereosinophilic syndrome in Hodgkin's disease with increased granulocyte-macrophage colony-stimulating factor. Ann Hematol 1995;71: 313–4.

[35] Jundt F, Anagnostopoulos I, Bommert K, et al. Hodgkin's/Reed-Sternberg cells induce fibroblasts to secrete eotaxin, a potent chemoattractant for T cells and eosinophils. Blood 1999;94(6):2065–71.

[36] Patella V, de Crescenzo G, Marino I, et al. Eosinophil granule proteins activate human heart mast cells. J Immunol 1996;157(3):1219–25.

[37] Pinto A, Aldinucci D, Gloghini A, et al. Human eosinophils express functional CD30 ligand and stimulate proliferation of a Hodgkin's disease cell line. Blood 1996;88(9): 3299–305.

[38] Kadin M, Butmarc J, Elovic A, et al. Eosinophils are the major source of transforming growth factor-beta 1 in nodular sclerosing Hodgkin's disease. Am J Pathol 1993;142(1):11–6.

[39] Newcom SR, Tagra KK. High molecular weight transforming growth factor beta is excreted in the urine in active nodular sclerosing Hodgkin's disease. Cancer Res 1992;52(24): 6768–73.

[40] Molin D, Glimelius B, Sundstrom C, et al. The serum levels of eosinophil cationic protein (ECP) are related to the infiltration of eosinophils in the tumours of patients with Hodgkin's disease. Leuk Lymphoma 2001;42(3):457–65.

[41] Hasenclever D, Diehl V. A prognostic score for advanced Hodgkin's disease. International prognostic factors project on advanced Hodgkin's Disease. N Engl J Med 1998;339(21): 1506–14.

[42] Fischer M, Harvima IT, Carvalho RF, et al. Mast cell CD30 ligand is upregulated in cutaneous inflammation and mediates degranulation-independent chemokine secretion. J Clin Invest 2006;116(10):2748–56.

[43] Salgami EV, Efstathiou SP, Vlachakis V, et al. High pretreatment interleukin-10 is an independent predictor of poor failure-free survival in patients with Hodgkin's lymphoma. Haematologia (Budap) 2002;32(4):377–87.

[44] Axdorph U, Sjoberg J, Grimfors G, et al. Biological markers may add to prediction of outcome achieved by the International Prognostic Score in Hodgkin's disease. Ann Oncol 2000;11(11):1405–11.

[45] Bohlen H, Kessler M, Sextro M, et al. Poor clinical outcome of patients with Hodgkin's disease and elevated interleukin-10 serum levels. Clinical significance of interleukin-10 serum levels for Hodgkin's disease. Ann Hematol 2000;79(3):110–3.

[46] Galli SJ, Nakae S, Tsai M. Mast cells in the development of adaptive immune response. Nat Immun 2005;6:135–42.

[47] Dimitriadou V, Koutsilieris M. Mast cell-tumor cell interactions: for or against tumour growth and metastasis? Anticancer Res 1997;17(3A):1541–9.

[48] Theoharides TC, Conti P. Mast cells: the Jekyll and Hyde of tumor growth. Trends Immunol 2004;25(5):235–41.

[49] Kirshenbaum AS, Goff JP, Semere T, et al. Demonstration that human mast cells arise from a progenitor cell population that is CD34(+), c-kit(+), and expresses aminopeptidase N (CD13). Blood 1999;94(7):2333–42.

[50] Galli SJ. Mast cells and basophils. Curr Opin Hematol 2000;7(1):32–9.

[51] Irani AA, Schechter NM, Craig SS, et al. Two types of human mast cells that have distinct neutral protease compositions. Proc Natl Acad Sci U S A 1986;83(12):4464–8.

[52] Coussens LM, Tinkle CL, Hanahan D, et al. MMP-9 supplied by bone marrow-derived cells contributes to skin carcinogenesis. Cell 2000;103(3):481–90.

[53] Ribatti D, Vacca A, Nico B, et al. The role of mast cells in tumour angiogenesis. Br J Haematol 2001;115(3):514–21.

[54] Glimelius I, Edstrom A, Fischer M, et al. Angiogenesis and mast cells in Hodgkin's lymphoma. Leukemia 2005;19(12):2360–2.

[55] Crocker J, Smith PJ. A quantitative study of mast cells in Hodgkin's disease. J Clin Pathol 1984;37(5):519–22.

[56] Sharma VK, Agrawal A, Pratap VK, et al. Mast cell reactivity in lymphoma: a preliminary communication. Indian J Cancer 1992;29(2):61–5.

[57] Levi-Schaffer F, Piliponsky AM. Tryptase, a novel link between allergic inflammation and fibrosis. Trends Immunol 2003;24(4):158–61.

[58] Teruya-Feldstein J, Tosato G, Jaffe ES. The role of chemokines in Hodgkin's disease. Leuk Lymphoma 2000;38(3–4):363–71.

[59] Teruya-Feldstein J, Jaffe ES, Burd PR, et al. Differential chemokine expression in tissues involved by Hodgkin's disease: direct correlation of eotaxin expression and tissue eosinophilia. Blood 1999;93(8):2463–70.

[60] Buri C, Korner M, Scharli P, et al. CC chemokines and the receptors CCR3 and CCR5 are differentially expressed in the nonneoplastic leukocytic infiltrates of Hodgkin's disease. Blood 2001;97(6):1543–8.

[61] Fischer M, Juremalm M, Olsson N, et al. Expression of CCL5/RANTES by Hodgkin's and Reed-Sternberg cells and its possible role in the recruitment of mast cells into lymphomatous tissue. Int J Cancer 2003;107(2):197–201.

[62] Nilsson G, Butterfield JH, Nilsson K, et al. Stem cell factor is a chemotactic factor for human mast cells. J Immunol 1994;153(8):3717–23.

[63] Juremalm M, Olsson N, Nilsson G. Selective CCL5/RANTES-induced mast cell migration through interactions with chemokine receptors CCR1 and CCR4. Biochem Biophys Res Commun 2002;297(3):480–5.

[64] Schwab U, Stein H, Gerdes J, et al. Production of a monoclonal antibody specific for Hodgkin's and Sternberg-Reed cells of Hodgkin's disease and a subset of normal lymphoid cells. Nature 1982;299(5878):65–7.

[65] Nawrocki JF, Kirsten ES, Fisher RI. Biochemical and structural properties of a Hodgkin's disease-related membrane protein. J Immunol 1988;141(2):672–80.

[66] Durkop H, Latza U, Hummel M, et al. Molecular cloning and expression of a new member of the nerve growth factor receptor family that is characteristic for Hodgkin's disease. Cell 1992;68(3):421–7.

[67] Gruss HJ, DaSilva N, Hu ZB, et al. Expression and regulation of CD30 ligand and CD30 in human leukemia-lymphoma cell lines. Leukemia 1994;8(12):2083–94.

[68] Josimovic-Alasevic O, Durkop H, Schwarting R, et al. Ki-1 (CD30) antigen is released by Ki-1-positive tumor cells in vitro and in vivo. I. Partial characterization of soluble Ki-1 antigen and detection of the antigen in cell culture supernatants and in serum by an enzyme-linked immunosorbent assay. Eur J Immunol 1989;19(1):157–62.

[69] Hansen HP, Kisseleva T, Kobarg J, et al. A zinc metalloproteinase is responsible for the release of CD30 on human tumor cell lines. Int J Cancer 1995;63(5):750–6.

[70] Gause A, Pohl C, Tschiersch A, et al. Clinical significance of soluble CD30 antigen in the sera of patients with untreated Hodgkin's disease. Blood 1991;77(9):1983–8.

[71] Zanotti R, Trolese A, Ambrosetti A, et al. Serum levels of soluble CD30 improve International Prognostic Score in predicting the outcome of advanced Hodgkin's lymphoma. Ann Oncol 2002;13(12):1908–14.

[72] Gruss HJ, Pinto A, Gloghini A, et al. CD30 ligand expression in nonmalignant and Hodgkin's disease-involved lymphoid tissues. Am J Pathol 1996;149(2):469–81.

[73] Wiley SR, Goodwin RG, Smith CA. Reverse signaling via CD30 ligand. J Immunol 1996;157(8):3635–9.

[74] Maggio E, van den Berg A, Diepstra A, et al. Chemokines, cytokines and their receptors in Hodgkin's lymphoma cell lines and tissues. Ann Oncol 2002;13(Suppl 1)):52–6.

[75] Skinnider BF, Mak TW. The role of cytokines in classical Hodgkin's lymphoma. Blood 2002;99(12):4283–97.

[76] Merz H, Houssiau FA, Orscheschek K, et al. Interleukin-9 expression in human malignant lymphomas: unique association with Hodgkin's disease and large cell anaplastic lymphoma. Blood 1991;78(5):1311–7.

[77] Erpenbeck VJ, Hohlfeld JM, Discher M, et al. Increased expression of interleukin-9 messenger RNA after segmental allergen challenge in allergic asthmatics. Chest 2003;123 (3 Suppl):370S.

[78] Knoops L, Renauld JC. IL-9 and its receptor: from signal transduction to tumorigenesis. Growth Factors 2004;22(4):207–15.

[79] Gruss HJ, Brach MA, Drexler HG, et al. Interleukin 9 is expressed by primary and cultured Hodgkin's and Reed-Sternberg cells. Cancer Res 1992;52(4):1026–31.

[80] Aldinucci D, Poletto D, Nanni P, et al. Hodgkin's and Reed-Sternberg cells express functional c-kit receptors and interact with primary fibroblasts from Hodgkin's disease-involved lymph nodes through soluble and membrane-bound stem cell factor. Br J Haematol 2002;118(4): 1055–64.

[81] Fischer M, Bijman M, Molin D, et-al. Increased serum levels of interleukin-9 correlate to negative prognostic factors in Hodgkin's lymphoma. Leukemia 2003;17(12):2513–6.

[82] Louahed J, Zhou Y, Maloy WL, et al. Interleukin 9 promotes influx and local maturation of eosinophils. Blood 2001;97(4):1035–42.

[83] Renauld JC, Kermouni A, Vink A, et al. Interleukin-9 and its receptor: involvement in mast cell differentiation and T cell oncogenesis. J Leukoc Biol 1995;57(3):353–60.

[84] Matsuzawa S, Sakashita K, Kinoshita T, et al. IL-9 enhances the growth of human mast cell progenitors under stimulation with stem cell factor. J Immunol 2003;170(7):3461–7.

[85] Aldinucci D, Lorenzon D, Olivo K, et al. Interactions between tissue fibroblasts in lymph nodes and Hodgkin's/Reed-Sternberg cells. Leuk Lymphoma 2004;45(9):1731–9.

[86] Folkman J. What is the evidence that tumors are angiogenesis dependent? J Natl Cancer Inst 1990;82(1):4–6.

[87] Korkolopoulou P TI, Kavantzas N, Vassilakopoulos TP, et al. Angiogenesis in Hodgkin's lymphoma: a morphometric approach in 286 patients with prognostic implications. Leukemia 2005;19(6):894–900.

[88] Mainou-Fowler T, Angus B, Miller S, et al. Micro-vessel density and the expression of vascular endothelial growth factor (VEGF) and platelet-derived endothelial cell growth factor (PdEGF) in classical Hodgkin's lymphoma (HL). Leuk Lymphoma 2006;47(2):223–30.

[89] Doussis-Anagnostopoulou IA, Talks KL, Turley H, et al. Vascular endothelial growth factor (VEGF) is expressed by neoplastic Hodgkin's-Reed-Sternberg cells in Hodgkin's disease. J Pathol 2002;197(5):677–83.

[90] Norrby K. Mast cells and angiogenesis. APMIS 2002;110(5):355–71.

[91] Carmeliet P. Angiogenesis in health and disease. Nat Med 2003;9(6):653–60.

[92] Gruss HJ, Herrmann F, Gattei V, et al. CD40/CD40 ligand interactions in normal, reactive and malignant lympho-hematopoietic tissues. Leuk Lymphoma 1997;24(5–6): 393–422.

[93] Hedvat CV, Jaffe ES, Qin J, et al. Macrophage-derived chemokine expression in classical Hodgkin's lymphoma: application of tissue microarrays. Mod Pathol 2001;14(12): 1270–6.

[94] Sanchez-Aguilera A, Montalban C, de la Cueva P, et al. Tumor microenvironment and mitotic checkpoint are key factors in the outcome of classic Hodgkin's lymphoma. Blood 2006;108(2):662–8.

[95] Grulich AE, Vajdic CM, Kaldor JM, et al. Birth order, atopy, and risk of non-Hodgkin's lymphoma. J Natl Cancer Inst 2005;97(8):587–94.

[96] Melbye M, Smedby KE, Lehtinen T, et al. Atopy and risk of non-Hodgkin's lymphoma. J Natl Cancer Inst 2007;99(2):158–66.

[97] Amlot PL, Slaney J, Brown R. Atopy–a favourable prognostic factor for survival in Hodgkin's disease. Br J Cancer 1983;48(2):209–15.

[98] Hogan SP, Foster PS. Cytokines as targets for the inhibition of eosinophilic inflammation. Pharmacol Ther 1997;74(3):259–83.

New Aspects in Descriptive, Etiologic, and Molecular Epidemiology of Hodgkin's Lymphoma

Ola Landgren, MD, PhD*, Neil E. Caporaso, MD

Genetic Epidemiology Branch, Division of Cancer Epidemiology and Genetics, National Cancer Institute, Department of Health and Human Services, National Institutes of Health, 6120 Executive Boulevard, Building EPS/Room 7110, Bethesda, MD 20892-7236, USA

H odgkin's disease was first described in 1832 by Thomas Hodgkin (1798–1866) who published his article entitled "On some morbid appearances of the adsorbent glands and spleen," describing the post-mortem appearance of seven patients who had enlargements of lymph nodes and spleen [1]. More than 30 years later, based on some 15 additional cases, Wilks published his article entitled "Cases of enlargement of the lymphatic glands and spleen, (or, Hodgkin's disease) with remarks" which ultimately named the disease after Thomas Hodgkin [2]. In 2001, the World Health Organization (WHO) lymphoma classification system designated Hodgkin's disease to Hodgkin's lymphoma [3].

Although Hodgkin's lymphoma is a rare hematopoietic malignancy in the general population [4,5], it has drawn much attention among generations of clinicians, pathologists, and researchers deriving from its generally unusual biology and epidemiology and because it is one of the first malignancies to exhibit curative response to chemotherapy. Its symptomatic features (such as recurrent cycles of fever, night sweats, and lymphadenopathy), which at times emerge clinically like an infectious disease, and preferential targeting of young adults have influenced many clinicians and researchers to suspect an infectious cause of the malignancy.

Etiologic clues about Hodgkin's lymphoma have been suggested by the bimodal age distribution; by elevated risks in males, in individuals with higher socioeconomic status, and in smaller families; and by the occurrence of Epstein-Barr virus in Hodgkin's lymphoma tumor cells [6,7]. After the introduction of highly active antiretroviral therapy (HAART) in 1996 for HIV-infected people, AIDS non-Hodgkin's lymphoma has declined substantially; however, the incidence of Hodgkin's lymphoma has been observed to increase simultaneously [8]. In the past decade, there have been reports showing increased

*Corresponding author. E-mail address: landgreo@mail.nih.gov (O. Landgren).

0889-8588/07/$ – see front matter
doi:10.1016/j.hoc.2007.07.001

Published by Elsevier Inc.
hemonc.theclinics.com

risk for Hodgkin's lymphoma among individuals who have undergone organ transplant or bone marrow transplant [9,10]. More recently, autoimmune and related conditions have drawn attention to a potential role for immune-related and inflammatory conditions in the cause and pathogenesis of the malignancy [11]. A role for genetic factors is unequivocal based on evidence from multiply affected families from case series, a twin study, a case-control study, and population-based registry studies [12–17]. Emerging data from Eastern Asia and among Chinese immigrants in North America indicate increasing incidence trends for Hodgkin's lymphoma associated with western-ization, which emphasizes the importance of lifestyle and environmental risk factors even in a short-term perspective [18,19].

CLASSIFICATIONS OF HODGKIN'S LYMPHOMA

Evolving Classification Systems

Jackson and Parker were the first to propose a comprehensive classification of Hodgkin's lymphoma [20,21]. This classification was subsequently found to be clinically irrelevant, because most of the patients belonged to the granuloma subtype with a huge variation in response to therapy and outcome. In 1956, Smetana and Cohen identified a variant of granuloma characterized by scle-rotic changes and a better prognosis [22]. Lukes and Butler suggested a histo-logic classification distinguishing six types of Hodgkin's lymphoma based on the varying degree of lymphocytic infiltration [23–25]. At the Rye symposium in 1965 the number of separate histologic groups was reduced from six to four and thereafter applied routinely for several decades because of the high repro-ducibility and good clinicopathologic correlations. In 1994, in light of morpho-logic, phenotypic, genotypic, and clinical findings, Hodgkin's lymphoma was listed in the Revised European-American Lymphoma classification and subdi-vided into two main types: nodular lymphocyte-predominant and classic Hodgkin's lymphoma [3,26]. Classic Hodgkin's lymphoma was further divided into four histologically and clinically defined subtypes: nodular sclerosis, mixed cellularity, lymphocyte-rich, and lymphocyte-depleted. This approach has been adopted by the most recent WHO classification of lymphomas [3], which promoted classic Hodgkin's lymphoma from a provisional to an accepted entity.

Heterogeneous Neoplastic Cells

Nodular lymphocyte-predominant and classic Hodgkin's lymphoma [3,26] share certain pathognomonic characteristics. For example, affected tissues con-tain only a small number of neoplastic Hodgkin's and Reed-Sternberg cells (typically less than 1%) in a background of nonneoplastic inflammatory and accessory cells [3], suggestive of a chronic inflammatory process. Several lines of evidence indicate that the neoplastic cells of Hodgkin's lymphoma originate from a germinal center or immediate postgerminal B cell that has been selected and stimulated by antigen [27–32]. Further, immunohistochemical studies have found neoplastic cells of nodular lymphocyte-predominant Hodgkin's lymphoma (popcorn cells) to be of BCL6+/CD138− phenotype, which is typical for germinal center cells. For the classic Hodgkin's lymphoma subtype, however, the neoplastic cells (Reed-Sternberg cells) have been observed to be typically BCL6+/CD138−, but sometimes they can be BCL6−/CD138+, which suggests that classic Hodgkin's lymphoma is a heterogeneous entity, including tumors of germinal center and postgerminal center B cell origin [33–35]. In rare cases of classic Hodgkin's lymphoma, tumor cells have been observed to be derived from peripheral (postthymic) T cells [36,37].

DESCRIPTIVE EPIDEMIOLOGY
Incidence and Mortality in Western Countries
Hodgkin's lymphoma composes about 11% of all lymphomas in western countries and has a unique bimodal (sometimes trimodal) age-incidence shape (Fig. 1). It is currently estimated by the American Cancer Society that there will be about 8190 new cases (55% males) and 1070 (72% males) deaths of Hodgkin's lymphoma in the United States in 2007 [38]. Also, the United States National Cancer Institute's Surveillance, Epidemiology, and End Results (SEER) and European-based International Agency for Research on Cancer

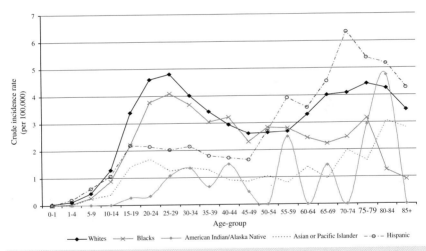

Fig. 1. Incidence of Hodgkin's lymphoma in the United States 1994–2003, by age and race. Statistics for American Indians/Alaska Natives do not include cases for the 2003 diagnosis year. Hispanic and Non-Hispanic are not mutually exclusive from White, Black, American Indian/Alaska Native, and Asian or Pacific Islander. Statistics for Hispanics and Non-Hispanics are based on NHIA and do not include cases from the Hawaii, Seattle, and Alaska Natives registries. Statistics for American Indians/Alaska Natives include cases from the Connecticut, Detroit, Iowa, New Mexico, Seattle, Utah, Atlanta and Alaska Natives registries. (*Data from* Surveillance, Epidemiology, and End Results (SEER) Program. SEER stat database: incidence—SEER13 regs public use, Nov 2005 Sub (1992–2003), National Cancer Institute, DCCPS, Surveillance Research Program, cancer Statistics branch, released April 2006, based on the November 2005 submission. Available at: http://www.seer.cancer.gov.)

population-based cancer registries have estimated the incidence of Hodgkin's lymphoma in the United States and in Europe to be around 2.3 to 3.1 per 100,000 males and 1.6 to 2.3 per 100,000 females, which underscores that Hodgkin's lymphoma is a rare malignancy in the general population [4,5]. Although the risk for developing Hodgkin's lymphoma is small (a life time risk of 0.24% for males and 0.20% for females) [5], it accounts for approximately 15% of all cancers in young adults (15 to 24 years). As to racial variation within the United States, a previous study on cancer incidence in California found the highest Hodgkin's lymphoma rates among whites, followed by African Americans and Hispanics, and the lowest incidence was observed among people of Asian descent [39]. This pattern is consistent with currently available data from the SEER database (see Fig. 1) [5].

The introduction of modern staging procedures and advances in radiotherapy and chemotherapy have significantly contributed to improved survival of patients who have Hodgkin's lymphoma over the past decades [40]. Clinical trials have observed long-term failure-free survival of 60% to 70% among patients treated with doxorubicin, bleomycin, vinblastine, and dacarbazine (ABVD)–based therapies [41,42]. The German Hodgkin's Study Group has reported further improved outcomes using their dose-escalated BEACOPP regimen (including cyclophosphamide, doxorubicin, etoposide, procarbazine, prednisone, vincristine, and bleomycin) developed for patients who have advanced-stage Hodgkin's lymphoma [43]. Consistent with results from clinical trials, data from 2000 to 2003 in the population-based SEER database reveal mortality rates for patients who have Hodgkin's lymphoma of 0.4 per 100,000 and 0.3 per 100,000 for males and females, respectively [5]. If one restricts the estimates to patients who are 65 years or older, the mortality rates are 2.1 per 100,000 (males) and 1.4 per 100,000 (females). By using 5-year relative survival rates as the measure of outcome the same pattern can be seen: the 5-year relative survival rates for all Hodgkin's lymphoma is about 85%, whereas the corresponding relative survival rate for older patients (65 years or older) is only 53% [5]. The outcomes of elderly (>50–60 years) patients still remain unsatisfactory, however, with inferior complete remission rates and overall survival [44–46]. Because older patients generally are not included in clinical trials the information on this topic is sparse. Population-based data from Scandinavia show that the 5-year overall survival for younger patients (diagnosed younger than age 50 years) increased from about 55% to 90% between the two calendar periods 1926 to 1955 and 1972 to 1994, whereas the corresponding improvement for patients diagnosed at 50 years or older improved from 20% to 50% during the same calendar periods [47,48]. Currently the underlying mechanisms for the clinically well-known poor prognosis of older patients who have Hodgkin's lymphoma treated with chemotherapy [49–53] remain unclear. Hodgkin's lymphoma in older patients is clinically more aggressive in that anemia, increased erythrocyte sedimentation rate, and B symptoms are significantly more frequent at diagnosis among the elderly [50,54], which supports the hypothesis of age-related disease differences in Hodgkin's lymphoma. Alternatively, aging itself and associated factors (such as increased comorbidity [55], reduced tolerability of conventional therapy [49,56], more severe toxicity and treatment-related deaths [57,58], and poorer outcome after relapse [59]) may contribute to the worse prognosis for elderly patients. Future research is needed to explore disease mechanisms by age for patients who have Hodgkin's lymphoma. Clinically, more accurate markers of outcome in combination with less toxic novel therapies are needed [44–46].

International Variation and Westernization

The incidence of Hodgkin's lymphoma has been found to vary between westernized countries versus economically disadvantaged countries (Fig. 2). In the early 1970s, three epidemiologic patterns were described by Correa and O'Conor: type I in developing countries (a first incidence peak in male children and a second peak in older age around 50 years, with a predominance of histopathologic subtypes mixed cellularity and lymphocyte-depleted); type II in rural areas of developed countries (an intermediate pattern with high male childhood incidence and a second decade peak among females); type III in developed urbanized countries (a bimodal age distribution with a pronounced peak in young adults experiencing nodular sclerosis as the most frequent histopathologic subtype, and a continuously rising incidence older than 40 years) [60]. Correa and O'Conor [60] suggested that the observed variation in international patterns of disease reflected differences in economic development (ie, correlated for example with the level of public hygiene). More recent data from the mid-1990s have shown that the incidence rates for young adults have increased in less developed countries while remaining static in western countries [61]. A recent study from Japan, where historically Hodgkin's lymphoma has been rare before the age of 50, reported increasing incidence of Hodgkin's lymphoma in recent decades [62]. The Cancer registry in Singapore has observed (in parallel with data from Hong Kong) that local rates of non-Hodgkin's lymphoma (1998–2002, n = 1170) are the highest in Asia and the incidence has steadily increased over the past four decades [19], consistent with the well-documented rising trends in western societies the past almost half century [63]. Between 1998 and 2002 the age-standardized rates for males and female were 8.2 and 5.0 per 100,000, respectively. During the period 1993–1997 the corresponding rates were 7.5 and 4.4 per 100,000 and for the period 1968–1972 they were 3.1 and 1.9, respectively. For Hodgkin's lymphoma, the number of cases between 1998 and 2002 is small (n = 122), making interpretation of the time trend difficult. There is evidence of an upward trend of the malignancy over the past decade, however [19].

In a recent study on incidence trends for Hodgkin's lymphoma among immigrants of Chinese descent in British Columbia, Canada, Au and colleagues [18] found the incidence of Hodgkin's lymphoma among Chinese immigrants to be significantly lower than expected from the British Columbia background population (standardized incidence ratio [SIR] = 0.34; $P <$ .0001). At the same

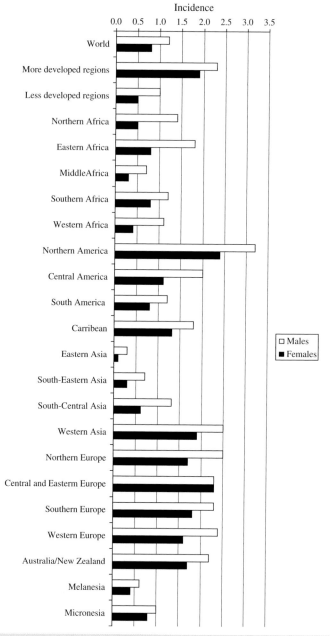

Fig. 2. Global incidence of Hodgkin's lymphoma 2002, by sex and region. Age-standardized rates per 100,000 person-years (world 2000 population). However, although the populations of the different countries are those estimated for the middle of 2002, the disease rates are not those for the year 2002, but from the most recent data available, generally 2–5 years earlier. The numbers of cases are computed by multiplying the estimated rates by the year 2002 population estimates for the corresponding country.The GLOBOCAN 2002 database provides estimates for the year 2002. (*Data from* Ferlay J, Bray F, Pisani P, et al. GLOBOCAN 2002: cancer incidence, mortality and prevalence worldwide. IARC CancerBase No. 5. version 2.0. Lyon: IARCPress; 2004.)

time, however, the incidence was significantly higher than that expected by extrapolating from the Hong Kong Chinese population (SIR = 2.81; $P < .0001$) [18]. The difference was mainly accounted for by young immigrants diagnosed with nodular sclerosis Hodgkin's lymphoma subtype. Although that study was restricted in size, it supports the hypothesis of a role for genetic, lifestyle, and environmental factors in the pathogenesis of Hodgkin's lymphoma. The results indicate that environmental and lifestyle factors can exert their influence over a relatively short period of time. Taken together, there is need for studies designed to quantify incidence trends for lymphomas in countries under the influence of westernization. Such results might provide opportunities to generate hypotheses regarding risk factors for the development of lymphomas and also are useful measures for health care planners who are responsible for future allocation of health care resources in these regions.

Secondary Tumors and Late Cardiovascular Disease
Developments in modern therapy have dramatically improved survival over the past decades for patients who have Hodgkin's lymphoma. Unfortunately, the improved outcome has been accompanied by long-term toxicity, such as elevated risk for second primary malignancies [64,65], cardiovascular disease [66], and infections [66,67]. In fact, second malignant neoplasms now are the leading cause of death among long-term survivors of Hodgkin's lymphoma [68], with breast cancer being the most common solid tumor among women [69]. The most pronounced risk for breast cancer has been found among women diagnosed with Hodgkin's lymphoma at age 30 years or younger [69–71] and is strongly associated with chest radiotherapy for Hodgkin's lymphoma. Risk has been reported to increase up to eightfold with increasing given radiation dose [69,71,72]. Other reported second cancers include acute nonlymphocytic leukemia, non-Hodgkin's lymphoma, lung cancer, stomach cancer, and melanoma [73]. Similar to the pattern of elevated risk for breast cancer, risks for other second cancer sites are highest among patients treated for Hodgkin's lymphoma at younger ages. Also, most solid tumors have been found to start within or at the edge of the irradiated field. Elevated radiation-related risks for second tumors have been found to increase even 20 to 30 years following therapy [73]. Finally, several studies have reported increased mortality of cardiac disease after mediastinal radiotherapy for Hodgkin's lymphoma [66,67]. Anthracycline chemotherapy significantly adds to the elevated risks of congestive heart failure (HR = 2.8) and valvular disorders (HR = 2.1) from mediastinal radiotherapy [74].

ETIOLOGIC AND MOLECULAR EPIDEMIOLOGY
Epstein-Barr Virus and Other Candidate Viruses
Over the past decades Epstein-Barr virus (EBV) has been the major candidate for an infectious agent causing Hodgkin's lymphoma. Previous studies have reported that individuals who have a personal history of infectious mononucleosis have an elevated risk for developing Hodgkin's lymphoma. The elevated risk for

Hodgkin's lymphoma has been found to be greater among people infected at older ages and weaker with time since infection [75]. Hypothetically, the observed association with infectious mononucleosis could reflect higher socioeconomic status resulting in relatively late infections with EBV. Based on Scandinavian data, however, there is no elevated risk for Hodgkin's lymphoma among first-degree relatives of patients who have infectious mononucleosis, strengthening the case for increased risk with infectious mononucleosis itself [75].

Previous studies investigating serum from patients who have Hodgkin's lymphoma have reported altered EBV antibody patterns. Typically, patients who have Hodgkin's lymphoma have higher mean antibody titers to EBV viral capsid antigen consistent with prior infection. Also, there is serologic evidence of elevated antibodies to early antigen and Epstein-Barr nuclear antigen among individuals subsequently diagnosed with Hodgkin's lymphoma [76].

Detection of the EBV genome has been reported in malignant cells of about one third to one half of the Hodgkin's lymphoma cases [76]. Almost all studies have demonstrated that EBV is more likely to be associated with the mixed cellularity subtype than with the nodular sclerosis subtype. The nodular lymphocyte-predominant subtype is not associated with EBV infection. The association of EBV with Hodgkin's lymphoma is strongest in children and the elderly and it is also more frequent in males than in females. The frequency of EBV association is higher in Asian and Central/Middle American countries than in the United States and Europe [77]. In situ hybridization and immunohistochemistry studies of affected tissues have demonstrated that EBV is localized to neoplastic Reed-Sternberg cells, which express EBV latent genes. Southern blot analysis of the fusion pattern of the EBV terminal repeat have shown that EBV in Reed-Sternberg cells is clonal. This evidence provides plausible evidence for the role of EBV in the pathogenesis of Hodgkin's lymphoma. EBV genome has only been found within the tumor in about 20% to 40% of patients who have Hodgkin's lymphoma with a prior diagnosis of infectious mononucleosis [78,79] and in around 30% to 40% of young adult patients overall [80]. Somewhat unexpected in relation to these findings, the association between infectious mononucleosis and Hodgkin's lymphoma has been found to be strongest for EBV-positive (versus EBV-negative) tumors [78,80]. One explanation is that EBV has been proposed to be the cause in patients who do not have viral genomic material within the tumor by way of a hit-and-run mechanism. Recent studies have not found evidence to support that hypothesis, however [81]. Based on the available evidence, the relationship between EBV and Hodgkin's lymphoma is plausible but unproven.

Several other viruses (such as cytomegalovirus, human herpesviruses 6, 7, and 8, polyoma viruses JC and BK, SV40, lymphotropic papovavirus, adenoviruses, human T-lymphotropic virus 1, and measles virus) have been examined as potential candidates or cofactors for involvement in Hodgkin's lymphoma. There is no consistent evidence indicating that these viruses are important in the cause of Hodgkin's lymphoma [82]. The risk for Hodgkin's lymphoma has been found to be elevated among people infected with HIV

[83]. Further, it has been observed that HIV-associated patients who have Hodgkin's lymphoma are more likely to be of mixed-cellularity or lymphocyte-depletion subtype and 80% to 100% of the cases have been reported to be EBV positive [84]. In a recent study investigating lymphoma trends in relation to HAART therapy, it was found that the dramatic decrease of non-Hodgkin's lymphoma has been paralleled by an increase of Hodgkin's lymphoma [8]. Currently, the underlying mechanisms for that observation remain unknown.

Autoimmunity and Hodgkin's Lymphoma

Autoimmune diseases are characterized by dysregulated lymphocyte reactivity against self-antigens and the production of autoantibodies, leading to damage of the targeted tissues, such as joints or skin [85]. Previous studies have shown that there is an increased risk for mainly non-Hodgkin's lymphoma subsequent to autoimmune conditions, including rheumatoid arthritis, Sjögren syndrome, and systemic lupus erythematosus [86–97]. Recent studies focusing on underlying pathophysiologic mechanisms related to lymphomagenesis have provided new evidence establishing differences in the risk for non-Hodgkin's lymphoma development associated with various autoimmune disorders [98]. A recent study investigated the association between a wide range of autoimmune conditions and subsequent risk for Hodgkin's lymphoma [11]. Elevated risk for Hodgkin's lymphoma was found for personal histories of several autoimmune conditions, including rheumatoid arthritis, systemic lupus erythematosus, sarcoidosis, and immune thrombocytopenic purpura. Also, a significant increased risk for Hodgkin's lymphoma was associated with family histories of sarcoidosis and ulcerative colitis. The association between personal and family history of sarcoidosis and a statistically significant increased risk for Hodgkin's lymphoma suggests shared susceptibility for these conditions.

Transplant and Hodgkin's Lymphoma

Allogeneic bone marrow transplantation is associated with an elevated risk for developing posttransplant lymphoproliferative disorders (PTLD). Although Hodgkin's lymphoma after transplantation is rare, an elevated risk has been reported [10]. Five of six assessable cases contained EBV genome. Differences from posttransplant lymphoproliferative disease after bone marrow transplantation were later onset (>2.5 years) and lack of association with established risk factors (such as T-cell depletion and human leukocyte antigen disparity). As pointed out by Rowlings and colleagues [10], the long latency of Hodgkin's lymphoma after transplant and the lack of association with risk factors for PTLD is remarkable and should be explored further for possible insights into pathogenesis.

Previous studies of solid organ transplant patients have not generally found an elevated risk for Hodgkin's lymphoma. The Israel Penn Transplant Tumor Registry lists Hodgkin's lymphoma as the lymphoid malignancy in 2.5% (31 cases) among 1252 diseases following solid organ transplant [99]. EBV nuclear material has been demonstrated in some of the cases of Hodgkin's lymphoma following transplantation [100,101].

Genetic Factors

The importance of genetic factors in Hodgkin's lymphoma is indicated by reports of multiply affected families from case series, a twin study, a case-control study, and population-based registry studies performed in Utah, Denmark, Israel, and Sweden [12–17]. Our group recently analyzed data from registries in Scandinavia and found significant familial aggregation of Hodgkin's lymphoma (relative risk = 3.1) and other lymphoproliferative tumors [13]. Relative risks were higher in males compared with females, and in siblings of patients compared with parents and offspring. Relatives of earlier-onset patients were at higher risk for Hodgkin's lymphoma and for all lymphoproliferative tumors and were also at higher risk for developing early onset tumors themselves.

Currently, it is not known whether (or how) extrinsic risk factors interact with genetic susceptibility. Identifying inherited susceptibility genes is an important step toward defining the pathways leading to development of Hodgkin's lymphoma and understanding its complex etiology. Until recently, there have been no comprehensive searches of the genome for Hodgkin's lymphoma genes, largely because of the difficulty in assembling informative samples. In 2005, a study including 44 informative high-risk Hodgkin's lymphoma families was conducted. In that study, whole-genome scanning was applied using densely spaced microsatellite markers to localize susceptibility genes [102]. The strongest linkage finding was on chromosome 4p near the marker D4S394. The logarithm of odds score calculated by Genehunter Plus was 2.6 (nominal $P = .0002$) when both Hodgkin's lymphoma and non-Hodgkin's lymphoma individuals were considered affected. Other locations suggestive of linkage were found on chromosomes 2 and 11. The findings from this investigation are consistent with recessive inheritance. These results are the first step in the discovery of germ line susceptibility genes and delineation of the pathways involved in development of Hodgkin's lymphoma. Future work is needed to better define pathways and to determine their interactions with environmental factors.

Other Factors

Based on the shape of the incidence curve for Hodgkin's lymphoma by age and gender, Glaser proposed in the mid-1990s that that childbearing potentially could be protective against Hodgkin's lymphoma in adult women [103]. Results from Norwegian studies have supported this hypothesis [104,105]; however, the difference in the shape of the incidence curves between the sexes was not seen in England and Wales [106].

Prior studies examining occupational exposures and subsequent cancer risk have reported on Hodgkin's lymphoma risk. The results on Hodgkin's lymphoma risk in relation to exposure to wood and wood dust and chemicals are inconsistent and based on small numbers. Phenoxy herbicides and chlorophenols have also been investigated but, again, there has not been consistent evidence of a causal association [107]. There is no evidence of an association of ionizing radiation with risk for Hodgkin's lymphoma. Some studies have found elevated risk for Hodgkin's lymphomas following tonsillectomy; however, the results are inconsistent.

FUTURE RESEARCH

Continued studies are needed to clarify the roles of EBV, HIV, and autoimmunity in the etiology and pathogenesis of Hodgkin's lymphoma. Future work also is needed to better define germ line susceptibility genes, to delineate pathways, and to determine their interactions with environmental factors. Observed increasing incidence trends for Hodgkin's lymphoma and their possible association with westernization should also be followed up.

Acknowledgments

This research was supported by the Intramural Research Program of the National Institutes of Health, National Cancer Institute.

References
[1] Hodgkin T. On some morbid experiences of the absorbent glands and spleen. Med Chir Trans 1832;17:69–97.
[2] Wilks S. Cases of enlargement of the lymphatic glands and spleen (or Hodgkin's disease), with remarks. Guy's Hosp Rep 1865;11:56–67.
[3] Jaffe ES, Harris NL, Stein H, Vardiman JW, editors. World Health Organization classification of tumours. Pathology and genetics of tumours of haematopoietic and lymphoid tissues. Lyon: IARC Press; 2001.
[4] Parkin DM, Whelan SL, Ferlay J, et al. Cancer incidence in five continents vol. I to VIII. Lyon: IARC; 2005 CancerBase No. 7.
[5] Ries LAG, Harkins D, Krapcho M, et al. SEER Cancer Statistics Review, 1975–2003. Bethesda, (MD): National Cancer Institute; 2006.
[6] O'Grady J, Stewart S, Elton RA, et al. Epstein-Barr virus in Hodgkin's disease and site of origin of tumour. Lancet 1994;343(8892):265–6.
[7] Diepstra A, Niens M, Vellenga E, et al. Association with HLA class I in Epstein-Barr-virus-positive and with HLA class III in Epstein-Barr-virus-negative Hodgkin's lymphoma. Lancet 2005;365(9478):2216–24.
[8] Biggar RJ, Jaffe ES, Goedert JJ, et al. Hodgkin lymphoma and immunodeficiency in persons with HIV/AIDS. Blood 2006;108(12):3786–91.
[9] Bierman PJ, Vose JM, Langnas AN, et al. Hodgkin's disease following solid organ transplantation. Ann Oncol 1996;7(3):265–70.
[10] Rowlings PA, Curtis RE, Passweg JR, et al. Increased incidence of Hodgkin's disease after allogeneic bone marrow transplantation. J Clin Oncol 1999;17(10):3122–7.
[11] Landgren O, Engels EA, Pfeiffer RM, et al. Autoimmunity and susceptibility to Hodgkin lymphoma: a population-based case-control study in Scandinavia. J Natl Cancer Inst 2006;98(18):1321–30.
[12] Goldgar DE, Easton DF, Cannon-Albright LA, et al. Systematic population-based assessment of cancer risk in first-degree relatives of cancer probands. J Natl Cancer Inst 1994;86(21):1600–8.
[13] Goldin LR, Pfeiffer RM, Gridley G, et al. Familial aggregation of Hodgkin lymphoma and related tumors. Cancer 2004;100(9):1902–8.
[14] Lindelof B, Eklund G. Analysis of hereditary component of cancer by use of a familial index by site. Lancet 2001;358(9294):1696–8.
[15] Paltiel O, Schmit T, Adler B, et al. The incidence of lymphoma in first-degree relatives of patients with Hodgkin disease and non-Hodgkin lymphoma: results and limitations of a registry-linked study. Cancer 2000;88(10):2357–66.

[16] Shugart YY, Hemminki K, Vaittinen P, et al. A genetic study of Hodgkin's lymphoma: an estimate of heritability and anticipation based on the familial cancer database in Sweden. Hum Genet 2000;106(5):553–6.

[17] Westergaard T, Melbye M, Pedersen JB, et al. Birth order, sibship size and risk of Hodgkin's disease in children and young adults: a population-based study of 31 million person-years. Int J Cancer 1997;72(6):977–81.

[18] Au WY, Gascoyne RD, Gallagher RE, et al. Hodgkin's lymphoma in Chinese migrants to British Columbia: a 25-year survey. Ann Oncol 2004;15(4):626–30.

[19] Seow A, Koh WP, Chia KS, et al. Trends in cancer incidence in Singapore 1968–2002. Singapore: Singapore Cancer Registry; 2004. p. 6.

[20] Jackson J, Parker J. Hodgkin's disease and allied disorders. New York: Oxford University Press; 1947.

[21] Harris NL. Hodgkin's lymphomas: classification, diagnosis, and grading. Semin Hematol 1999;36(3):220–32.

[22] Smetana HF, Cohen BM. Mortality in relation to histologic type in Hodgkin's disease. Blood 1956;11(3):211–24.

[23] Rosenthal S. Significance of tissue lymphocytes in the prognosis of lymphogranulomatosis. Arch Pathol 1936;21:628–46.

[24] Lukes RJ. Relationship of histologic features to clinical stages in Hodgkin's disease. Am J Roentgenol Radium Ther Nucl Med 1963;90:944–55.

[25] Lukes RJ, Butler JJ. The pathology and nomenclature of Hodgkin's disease. Cancer Res 1966;26(6):1063–83.

[26] Harris NL, Jaffe ES, Diebold J, et al. Lymphoma classification—from controversy to consensus: the R.E.A.L. and WHO Classification of lymphoid neoplasms. Ann Oncol 2000;11(Suppl 1): 3–10.

[27] Cossman J, Annunziata CM, Barash S, et al. Reed-Sternberg cell genome expression supports a B-cell lineage. Blood 1999;94(2):411–6.

[28] Brauninger A, Hansmann ML, Strickler JG, et al. Identification of common germinal-center B-cell precursors in two patients with both Hodgkin's disease and non-Hodgkin's lymphoma. N Engl J Med 1999;340(16):1239–47.

[29] Kuppers R, Roers A, Kanzler H. Molecular single cell studies of normal and transformed lymphocytes. Cancer Surv 1997;30:45–58.

[30] Marafioti T, Hummel M, Anagnostopoulos I, et al. Origin of nodular lymphocyte-predominant Hodgkin's disease from a clonal expansion of highly mutated germinal-center B cells. N Engl J Med 1997;337(7):453–8.

[31] Marafioti T, Hummel M, Foss HD, et al. Hodgkin and Reed-Sternberg cells represent an expansion of a single clone originating from a germinal center B-cell with functional immunoglobulin gene rearrangements but defective immunoglobulin transcription. Blood 2000;95(4):1443–50.

[32] Braeuninger A, Kuppers R, Strickler JG, et al. Hodgkin and Reed-Sternberg cells in lymphocyte predominant Hodgkin disease represent clonal populations of germinal center-derived tumor B cells. Proc Natl Acad Sci U S A 1997;94(17):9337–42.

[33] Falini B, Mason DY. Proteins encoded by genes involved in chromosomal alterations in lymphoma and leukemia: clinical value of their detection by immunocytochemistry. Blood 2002;99(2):409–26.

[34] Carbone A, Gloghini A, Gaidano G, et al. Expression status of BCL-6 and syndecan-1 identifies distinct histogenetic subtypes of Hodgkin's disease. Blood 1998;92(7): 2220–8.

[35] Falini B, Bigerna B, Pasqualucci L, et al. Distinctive expression pattern of the BCL-6 protein in nodular lymphocyte predominance Hodgkin's disease. Blood 1996;87(2): 465–71.

[36] Muschen M, Rajewsky K, Brauninger A, et al. Rare occurrence of classical Hodgkin's disease as a T cell lymphoma. J Exp Med 2000;191(2):387–94.

[37] Seitz V, Hummel M, Marafioti T, et al. Detection of clonal T-cell receptor gamma-chain gene rearrangements in Reed-Sternberg cells of classic Hodgkin disease. Blood 2000;95(10): 3020–4.

[38] Anonymous. Cancer facts & figures 2007. Atlanta (GA): American Cancer Society; 2007.

[39] Perkins CI, Morris CR, Wright WE, et al. Cancer incidence and mortality in California by detailed race/ethnicity, 1988–1992. Sacramento (CA): California Department of Health Services Surveillance Section; 1995.

[40] Kennedy BJ, Fremgen AM, Menck HR. The National Cancer Data Base report on Hodgkin's disease for 1985–1989 and 1990–1994. Cancer 1998;83(5):1041–7.

[41] Duggan DB, Petroni GR, Johnson JL, et al. Randomized comparison of ABVD and MOPP/ ABV hybrid for the treatment of advanced Hodgkin's disease: report of an intergroup trial. J Clin Oncol 2003;21(4):607–14.

[42] Canellos GP, Anderson JR, Propert KJ, et al. Chemotherapy of advanced Hodgkin's disease with MOPP, ABVD, or MOPP alternating with ABVD. N Engl J Med 1992;327(21): 1478–84.

[43] Diehl V, Behringer K. Could BEACOPP be the new standard for the treatment of advanced Hodgkin's lymphoma (HL)? Cancer Invest 2006;24(7):713–7.

[44] Forsyth PD, Bessell EM, Moloney AJ, et al. Hodgkin's disease in patients older than 70 years of age: a registry-based analysis. Eur J Cancer 1997;33(10):1638–42.

[45] Eghbali H, Hoerni-Simon G, de Mascarel I, et al. Hodgkin's disease in the elderly. A series of 30 patients aged older than 70 years. Cancer 1984;53(10):2191–3.

[46] Wedelin C, Bjorkholm M, Biberfeld P, et al. Prognostic factors in Hodgkin's disease with special reference to age. Cancer 1984;53(5):1202–8.

[47] Landgren O. Diagnostic and prognostic studies in Hodgkin's lymphoma. Stockholm: Department of Medicine, Division of Hematology, Karolinska Institutet; 2002.

[48] Westling P. Studies of the prognosis in Hodgkin's disease. Acta Radiol 1965;(Suppl 245): 5–125.

[49] Landgren O, Algernon C, Axdorph U, et al. Hodgkin's lymphoma in the elderly with special reference to type and intensity of chemotherapy in relation to prognosis. Haematologica 2003;88(4):438–44.

[50] Engert A, Ballova V, Haverkamp H, et al. Hodgkin's lymphoma in elderly patients: a comprehensive retrospective analysis from the German Hodgkin's Study Group. J Clin Oncol 2005;23(22):5052–60.

[51] Ballova V, Ruffer JU, Haverkamp H, et al. A prospectively randomized trial carried out by the German Hodgkin Study Group (GHSG) for elderly patients with advanced Hodgkin's disease comparing BEACOPP baseline and COPP-ABVD (study HD9elderly). Ann Oncol 2005;16(1):124–31.

[52] Weekes CD, Vose JM, Lynch JC, et al. Hodgkin's disease in the elderly: improved treatment outcome with a doxorubicin-containing regimen. J Clin Oncol 2002;20(4): 1087–93.

[53] Proctor SJ, White J, Jones GL. An international approach to the treatment of Hodgkin's disease in the elderly: launch of the SHIELD study programme. Eur J Haematol Suppl 2005;(66):63–7.

[54] Landgren O, Axdorph U, Fears TR, et al. A population-based cohort study on early-stage Hodgkin lymphoma treated with radiotherapy alone: with special reference to older patients. Ann Oncol 2006;17(8):1290–5.

[55] van Spronsen DJ, Janssen-Heijnen ML, Breed WP, et al. Prevalence of co-morbidity and its relationship to treatment among unselected patients with Hodgkin's disease and non-Hodgkin's lymphoma, 1993–1996. Ann Hematol 1999;78(7):315–9.

[56] Erdkamp FL, Breed WP, Bosch LJ, et al. Hodgkin disease in the elderly. A registry-based analysis. Cancer 1992;70(4):830–4.

[57] Peterson BA, Pajak TF, Cooper MR, et al. Effect of age on therapeutic response and survival in advanced Hodgkin's disease. Cancer Treat Rep 1982;66(4):889–98.

[58] Levis A, Depaoli L, Bertini M, et al. Results of a low aggressivity chemotherapy regimen (CVP/CEB) in elderly Hodgkin's disease patients. Haematologica 1996;81(5):450–6.

[59] Specht L, Nissen NI. Hodgkin's disease and age. Eur J Haematol 1989;43(2):127–35.

[60] Correa P, O'Conor GT. Epidemiologic patterns of Hodgkin's disease. Int J Cancer 1971;8(2):192–201.

[61] Macfarlane GJ, Evstifeeva T, Boyle P, et al. International patterns in the occurrence of Hodgkin's disease in children and young adult males. Int J Cancer 1995;61(2):165–9.

[62] Aozasa K, Ueda T, Tamai M, et al. Hodgkin's disease in Osaka, Japan (1964–1985). Eur J Cancer Clin Oncol 1986;22(9):1117–9.

[63] Clarke CA, Glaser SL. Changing incidence of non-Hodgkin lymphomas in the United States. Cancer 2002;94(7):2015–23.

[64] Ng AK, Bernardo MV, Weller E, et al. Second malignancy after Hodgkin disease treated with radiation therapy with or without chemotherapy: long-term risks and risk factors. Blood 2002;100(6):1989–96.

[65] Dores GM, Metayer C, Curtis RE, et al. Second malignant neoplasms among long-term survivors of Hodgkin's disease: a population-based evaluation over 25 years. J Clin Oncol 2002;20(16):3484–94.

[66] Ng AK, Bernardo MP, Weller E, et al. Long-term survival and competing causes of death in patients with early-stage Hodgkin's disease treated at age 50 or younger. J Clin Oncol 2002;20(8):2101–8.

[67] Aleman BM, van den Belt-Dusebout AW, Klokman WJ, et al. Long-term cause-specific mortality of patients treated for Hodgkin's disease. J Clin Oncol 2003;21(18):3431–9.

[68] Hoppe RT. Hodgkin's disease: complications of therapy and excess mortality. Ann Oncol 1997;8(Suppl 1):115–8.

[69] Travis LB, Hill DA, Dores GM, et al. Breast cancer following radiotherapy and chemotherapy among young women with Hodgkin disease. JAMA 2003;290(4):465–75.

[70] van Leeuwen FE, Klokman WJ, Stovall M, et al. Roles of radiation dose, chemotherapy, and hormonal factors in breast cancer following Hodgkin's disease. J Natl Cancer Inst 2003;95(13):971–80.

[71] Hill DA, Gilbert E, Dores GM, et al. Breast cancer risk following radiotherapy for Hodgkin lymphoma: modification by other risk factors. Blood 2005;106(10):3358–65.

[72] Travis LB, Hill D, Dores GM, et al. Cumulative absolute breast cancer risk for young women treated for Hodgkin lymphoma. J Natl Cancer Inst 2005;97(19):1428–37.

[73] Foss Abrahamsen A, Andersen A, Nome O, et al. Long-term risk of second malignancy after treatment of Hodgkin's disease: the influence of treatment, age and follow-up time. Ann Oncol 2002;13(11):1786–91.

[74] Aleman BM, van den Belt-Dusebout AW, De Bruin ML, et al. Late cardiotoxicity after treatment for Hodgkin lymphoma. Blood 2007;109(5):1878–86.

[75] Hjalgrim H, Askling J, Sorensen P, et al. Risk of Hodgkin's disease and other cancers after infectious mononucleosis. J Natl Cancer Inst 2000;92(18):1522–8.

[76] Mueller NE. Hodgkin's disease. In: Schottenfeld D, Fraumeni JF Jr, editors. Cancer epidemiology and prevention. 2nd edition. New York: Oxford University Press; 1996. p. 893–919.

[77] Tomita Y, Ohsawa M, Kanno H, et al. Epstein-Barr virus in Hodgkin's disease patients in Japan. Cancer 1996;77(1):186–92.

[78] Alexander FE, Jarrett RF, Lawrence D, et al. Risk factors for Hodgkin's disease by Epstein-Barr virus (EBV) status: prior infection by EBV and other agents. Br J Cancer 2000;82(5): 1117–21.

[79] Sleckman BG, Mauch PM, Ambinder RF, et al. Epstein-Barr virus in Hodgkin's disease: correlation of risk factors and disease characteristics with molecular evidence of viral infection. Cancer Epidemiol Biomarkers Prev 1998;7(12):1117–21.

[80] Glaser SL, Lin RJ, Stewart SL, et al. Epstein-Barr virus-associated Hodgkin's disease: epidemiologic characteristics in international data. Int J Cancer 1997;70(4):375–82.

[81] Gallagher A, Perry J, Freeland J, et al. Hodgkin lymphoma and Epstein-Barr virus (EBV): no evidence to support hit-and-run mechanism in cases classified as non-EBV-associated. Int J Cancer 2003;104(5):624–30.

[82] Benharroch D, Shemer-Avni Y, Levy A, et al. New candidate virus in association with Hodgkin's disease. Leuk Lymphoma 2003;44(4):605–10.

[83] Goedert JJ, Cote TR, Virgo P, et al. Spectrum of AIDS-associated malignant disorders. Lancet 1998;351(9119):1833–9.

[84] Carbone A, Gloghini A. AIDS-related lymphomas: from pathogenesis to pathology. Br J Haematol 2005;130(5):662–70.

[85] Klippel JH. Primer on the rheumatic diseases. 12th edition. Atlanta (GA): Arthritis Foundation; 2001.

[86] Bjornadal L, Lofstrom B, Yin L, et al. Increased cancer incidence in a Swedish cohort of patients with systemic lupus erythematosus. Scand J Rheumatol 2002;31(2):66–71.

[87] Kassan SS, Thomas TL, Moutsopoulos HM, et al. Increased risk of lymphoma in sicca syndrome. Ann Intern Med 1978;89(6):888–92.

[88] Isomaki HA, Hakulinen T, Joutsenlahti U. Excess risk of lymphomas, leukemia and myeloma in patients with rheumatoid arthritis. J Chronic Dis 1978;31(11):691–6.

[89] Mellemkjaer L, Andersen V, Linet MS, et al. Non-Hodgkin's lymphoma and other cancers among a cohort of patients with systemic lupus erythematosus. Arthritis Rheum 1997;40(4):761–8.

[90] Gridley G, McLaughlin JK, Ekbom A, et al. Incidence of cancer among patients with rheumatoid arthritis. J Natl Cancer Inst 1993;85(4):307–11.

[91] Ekstrom K, Hjalgrim H, Brandt L, et al. Risk of malignant lymphomas in patients with rheumatoid arthritis and in their first-degree relatives. Arthritis Rheum 2003;48(4):963–70.

[92] Thomas E, Brewster DH, Black RJ, et al. Risk of malignancy among patients with rheumatic conditions. Int J Cancer 2000;88(3):497–502.

[93] Mellemkjaer L, Alexander F, Olsen JH. Cancer among children of parents with autoimmune diseases. Br J Cancer 2000;82(7):1353–7.

[94] Hartge P, Wang SS. Overview of the etiology and epidemiology of lymphoma. In: Mauch P, Armitage J, Lee N, Dalla-Favera R, Coiffier B, editors. Non-Hodgkin's lymphoma. Philadelphia: Lippincott Williams & Wilkins; 2004.

[95] Landgren O, Kerstann KF, Gridley G, et al. Re: Familial clustering of Hodgkin lymphoma and multiple sclerosis. J Natl Cancer Inst 2005;97(7):543–4.

[96] Smedby KE, Hjalgrim H, Askling J, et al. Autoimmune and chronic inflammatory disorders and risk of non-Hodgkin lymphoma by subtype. J Natl Cancer Inst 2006;98(1):51–60.

[97] Engels EA, Cerhan JR, Linet MS, et al. Immune-related conditions and immune-modulating medications as risk factors for non-Hodgkin's lymphoma: a case-control study. Am J Epidemiol 2005;162(12):1153–61.

[98] Zintzaras E, Voulgarelis M, Moutsopoulos HM. The risk of lymphoma development in autoimmune diseases: a meta-analysis. Arch Intern Med 2005;165(20):2337–44.

[99] Penn I. Neoplastic complications of transplantation. Semin Respir Infect 1993;8(3):233–9.

[100] Haluska FG, Brufsky AM, Canellos GP. The cellular biology of the Reed-Sternberg cell. Blood 1994;84(4):1005–19.

[101] Garnier JL, Lebranchu Y, Lefrancois N, et al. Hodgkin's disease after renal transplantation. Transplant Proc 1995;27(2):1785.

[102] Goldin LR, McMaster ML, Ter-Minassian M, et al. A genome screen of families at high risk for Hodgkin lymphoma: evidence for a susceptibility gene on chromosome 4. J Med Genet 2005;42(7):595–601.

[103] Glaser SL. Reproductive factors in Hodgkin's disease in women: a review. Am J Epidemiol 1994;139(3):237–46.

[104] Kravdal O, Hansen S. The importance of childbearing for Hodgkin's disease: new evidence from incidence and mortality models. Int J Epidemiol 1996;25(4):737–43.

[105] Kravdal O, Hansen S. Hodgkin's disease: the protective effect of childbearing. Int J Cancer 1993;55(6):909–14.

[106] Swerdlow A, dos Santos Silva I, Doll R. Cancer incidence and mortality in England and Wales: trends and risk factors. Oxford (UK): Oxford University Press; 2001.

[107] McCunney RJ. Hodgkin's disease, work, and the environment. A review. J Occup Environ Med 1999;41(1):36–46.

The International Harmonization Project for Response Criteria in Lymphoma Clinical Trials

Bruce D. Cheson, MD

Georgetown University Hospital, 3800 Reservoir Road, NW, Washington, DC 20007 USA

C linical trials are critical to the development of newer and more effective treatments. Standardized response criteria are essential to assess and compare the activity of various therapies within and among studies and to facilitate the evaluation of new treatments by regulatory agencies. Even minor differences in response criteria, such as the size of a lymph node to be considered normal, can have a major impact on the level of interest in a new drug [1]. In 1999, an international working group (IWG) of clinicians, radiologists, and pathologists with expertise in the evaluation and management of patients who have lymphoma developed guidelines that codified the size of a normal lymph node and when and how responses were assessed, and provided definitions for the terms complete remission (CR), complete remission unconfirmed (CRu), Partial remission (PR), stable disease (SD), relapse (RD), and progressive disease (PD) [2]. These recommendations were rapidly and widely accepted by clinicians and regulatory agencies and, although initially intended for non-Hodgkin's lymphoma, were soon incorporated into Hodgkin's lymphoma studies also.

As these criteria were used over the next few years, several issues became apparent that warranted their reassessment. For example, the IWG criteria relied on physical examination, with its marked inter- and intraobserver variability, CT scans, and SPECT gallium scans, the latter no longer being widely used.

Another problem with the original IWG criteria was that several the features were misinterpreted. For example, CRu was originally proposed to specify two types of responses to treatment: the first group included those patients who had potentially curable tumors, such as Hodgkin's lymphoma and diffuse large B-cell lymphoma (DLBCL), for whom treatment resulted in disappearance of all detectable tumor with the exception of a single mass that decreased by at least 75% on CT scan but was still present. Numerous studies had previously

E-mail address: bdc4@georgetown.edu

0889-8588/07/$ – see front matter
doi:10.1016/j.hoc.2007.06.011
© 2007 Elsevier Inc. All rights reserved.
hemonc.theclinics.com

demonstrated that in as many as 90% of cases these lesions represented scar tissue or fibrosis [3,4]. Instead, the designation CRu was often applied to partial responses with a decrease in the sum of the product of the diameters (SPD) of multiple nodes by at least 75%, even in patients who had incurable histologies. The result was that the CR rate was artificially inflated. The second type of CRu included patients who had bone marrow involvement before treatment who fulfilled all of the conditions for a CR following therapy except that re-biopsy of the bone marrow was considered by the pathologist to be morphologically indeterminate. Instead, the term was also assigned to patients who did not undergo a confirmatory rebiopsy.

One of the most compelling arguments for revising the IWG criteria was the increased availability of newer and more sensitive technologies. The most notable of these are 18-fluorodeoxyglucose (FDG) positron emission tomography (PET) scanning, immunohistochemistry, and flow cytometry. Each of these tests has improved the ability to distinguish lymphoma from normal tissue, reducing the inter- and intraobserver variability and bias encountered with previous techniques.

PET is being increasingly used for staging, restaging, and response assessment of lymphomas [5–28]. PET is superior to CT in its ability to distinguish between viable tumor and necrosis or fibrosis in residual masses following treatment, which may have important clinical implications [10,12,29–31]. Juweid and colleagues [21] were the first to demonstrate how integrating PET into the IWG criteria in patients who had diffuse large B-cell non-Hodgkin's lymphoma not only increased the number of patients categorized as a CR but also eliminated the category of CRu and provided an enhanced discrimination in progression-free survival of CR and PR patients.

Nevertheless, several important limitations of PET remained to be resolved. There were important differences in equipment technique and variability in interpretation among readers. Histologic subtypes differ in their FDG avidity [11,32–35]. Moreover, there are many common causes of false-positive and false-negative PET scans [20,27,33,36,37].

In 2005, the German Competence Network Malignant Lymphoma evaluated compliance with the IWG criteria among nine lymphoma study groups and identified numerous discrepancies [38]. As a consequence, the International Harmonization Project convened an international committee of lymphoma investigators, pathologists, and nuclear medicine physicians to review the IWG and other proposed response criteria (eg, RECIST) and to modify and update them to ensure consistency among international study groups. A series of meetings were held and subcommittees were formed to focus on clinical features, pathology, imaging, and study endpoints.

The International Harmonization subcommittees developed their consensus reports that were recently published as revised guidelines. The first standardized the performance and interpretation of PET in lymphoma clinical trials [27]. The second was a revision of the response criteria incorporating of PET, immunohistochemistry, and flow cytometry [28].

THE USE OF POSITRON EMISSION TOMOGRAPHY IN CLINICAL TRIALS

The recommendations concerning the use of PET scans reflected the variability in FDG avidity among the various lymphoma histologic subtypes, and the relevant endpoints of the clinical trial (Table 1). For example, for patients who had routinely FDG-avid, potentially curable lymphomas (eg, DLBCL, Hodgkin's lymphoma) PET is strongly recommended before treatment to better delineate the extent of disease and to provide a baseline for posttreatment comparisons; however, PET was not mandated because of current limitations imposed by cost and availability. For the incurable histologies that are FDG-avid (eg, follicular, low-grade, and mantle cell lymphoma) and those histologies that are variable in their FDG avidity, PET is not recommended before treatment unless response rate, particularly complete response, is a primary endpoint of the trial because time-dependent endpoints (eg, progression-free survival) are often of greater importance.

Although numerous studies have demonstrated that the results of PET scans performed after one or more cycles of chemotherapy correlate with progression-free and overall survival [6–8,22,25,39,40], there are no data that demonstrate an improvement in clinical outcome by altering treatment on the basis of these results. This issue remains one of the most important questions in lymphoma therapy and is currently being addressed in several studies.

PET was considered essential for restaging of the curable lymphoma histologies following completion of therapy, because a complete remission is a prerequisite for cure and therapeutic intervention is generally warranted if residual disease is present. PET is not recommended in the posttreatment assessment of incurable histologies, however, unless the PET scan was positive before

Table 1
Recommended timing of PET/CT scans in lymphoma clinical trials

Histology	Pretreatment	Midtreatment	Response assessment	Posttreatment surveillance
Routinely FDG-avid				
DLBCL	Yes[a]	Clinical trial	Yes	No
HL	Yes[a]	Clinical trial	Yes	No
Follicular NHL	No[b]	Clinical trial	No[b]	No
MCL	No[b]	Clinical trial	No[b]	No
Variably FDG-avid				
Other aggressive NHLs	No[b]	Clinical trial	No[b,c]	No
Other indolent NHLs	No[b]	Clinical trial	No[b,c]	No

Abbreviations: DLBCL, diffuse large B-cell lymphoma; Hodgkin's lymphoma; MCL, mantle cell lymphoma; NHL, non-Hodgkin's lymphoma
  [a]Recommended but not required pretreatment.
  [b]Recommended only if overall response rate/CR is a primary study endpoint.
  [c]Recommended only if PET is positive pretreatment.
  Data from Cheson BD, Pfistner B, Juweid ME, et al. Revised response criteria for malignant lymphoma. J Clin Oncol 2007;25:579–86.

treatment and if complete response rate is a primary endpoint of a clinical study.

The timing of PET scans following the completion of treatment is important. In general, PET scans should not be performed until at least 3 weeks, and preferably 6 to 8 weeks, following completion of therapy to reduce the likelihood of a false-positive result [27]. Nevertheless, the use of PET for the early assessment of response for new drug development is a subject of considerable research interest [41]. A complete review of the current recommendations for PET interpretation is beyond the scope of this article and can be found in the recent publication by the International Harmonization Project [27]. In summary, positive scan has been defined as focal or diffuse FDG uptake above background in a location incompatible with normal anatomy or physiology. The numerous causes of false-positive scans must be ruled out, however [37]. Exceptions include mild and diffusely increased FDG uptake at the site of moderate- or large-sized masses with an intensity that is lower than or equal to the mediastinal blood pool, hepatic or splenic nodules 1.5 cm with FDG uptake lower than the surrounding liver/spleen uptake, and diffusely increased bone marrow uptake within weeks following treatment [27]. Areas of necrosis may be FDG-avid within an otherwise negative residual mass and a follow-up scan in a few months is often indicated to confirm this clinical impression. Visual assessment is currently considered adequate for determining whether a PET scan is positive, and using the standardized uptake value (SUV) is not necessary [27]. What proportion of a reduction in SUV correlates with response is currently being evaluated.

Given these considerations, the new IWG response criteria were developed to incorporate PET (Table 2).

REVISED RESPONSE CRITERIA
Complete Remission
Complete remission requires:

> Complete disappearance of all clinical evidence of disease and disease-related symptoms.

a. Typically FDG-avid lymphoma: In patients who had no pretreatment PET scan or when the FDG-PET scan was positive before therapy a posttreatment residual mass of any size is permitted as long as it is PET-negative.

b. Variably FDG-avid lymphomas/FDG avidity unknown: In patients who had no pretreatment PET scan, or if a pretreatment PET scan was negative all lymph nodes and nodal masses must have regressed on CT to normal size ($\leq$1.5 cm in their greatest transverse diameter for nodes >1.5 cm before therapy). Previously involved nodes that were 1.1 to 1.5 cm in their long axis and >1.0 cm in their short axis before treatment must have decreased to $\leq$1.0 cm in their short axis after treatment.

> The spleen and/or liver, if considered enlarged before therapy on the basis of a physical examination or CT scan, should not be palpable on physical examination and should be considered normal size by imaging studies, and

nodules related to lymphoma should disappear. Determination of splenic involvement is not always reliable, however, because a spleen considered normal in size may still contain lymphoma, whereas an enlarged spleen may reflect variations in anatomy, blood volume, the use of hematopoietic growth factors, or causes other than lymphoma.

If the bone marrow was involved by lymphoma before treatment, the infiltrate must have cleared on repeat bone marrow biopsy. The biopsy sample on which this determination is made must be adequate (with a goal of >20 mm unilateral core). If the sample is indeterminate by morphology, it should be negative by immunohistochemistry. A sample that is negative by immunohistochemistry but demonstrating a small population of clonal lymphocytes by flow cytometry is considered a CR until data become available demonstrating a clear difference in patient outcome.

Complete Remission/Unconfirmed

Using the above definition for CR and that below for PR eliminates the category of CRu.

Partial Remission

Partial remission requires all of the following:

A ≥50% decrease in sum of the product of the diameters (SPD) of up to six of the largest dominant nodes or nodal masses. These nodes or masses should be selected according to all of the following: (a) they should be clearly measurable in at least two perpendicular dimensions; (b) if possible, they should be from disparate regions of the body; (c) they should include mediastinal and retroperitoneal areas of disease whenever these sites are involved.

No increase in the size of other nodes, liver, or spleen.

Splenic and hepatic nodules must regress by ≥50% in their SPD or, for single nodules, in the greatest transverse diameter.

With the exception of splenic and hepatic nodules, involvement of other organs is usually evaluable and not measurable disease.

Bone marrow assessment is irrelevant for determination of a PR if the sample was positive before treatment. If positive, the cell type should be specified (eg, large cell lymphoma or small neoplastic B cells). Patients who achieve a complete remission by the above criteria, but who have persistent morphologic bone marrow involvement, are considered partial responders. For cases in which the bone marrow was involved before therapy that resulted in a clinical CR, but with no bone marrow assessment following treatment, patients should be considered partial responders.

No new sites of disease.

Typically FDG-avid lymphoma: For patients who had no pretreatment PET scan or if the PET scan was positive before therapy, the posttreatment PET should be positive in at least one previously involved site.

Variably FDG-avid lymphomas/FDG-avidity unknown: For patients who had no pretreatment PET scan, or if a pretreatment PET scan was negative, CT criteria should be used.

Table 2
Response definitions for clinical trials

Response	Definition	Nodal masses	Spleen, liver	Bone marrow
Complete remission (CR)	Disappearance of all evidence of diseases	a. FDG-avid or PET+ before therapy: mass of any size permitted if PET− b. Variably FDG-avid or PET−: regression to normal size on CT	Not palpable, nodules disappeared	Infiltrate cleared on repeat biopsy; if indeterminate by morphology, immunohistochemistry should be negative
Partial remission (PR)	Regression of measurable disease and no new sites	≥50% decrease in SPD of up to six largest dominant masses. No increase in size of other nodes a. FDG-avid or PET+ before therapy: one or more PET+ at previously involved site b. Variably FDG-avid or PET−: regression on CT	≥50% decrease in SPD of nodules (for single nodule in greatest transverse diameter) no increase in size of liver or spleen	Irrelevant if positive before therapy; cell type should be specified
Stable disease (SD)	Failure to attain CR/PR or PD	a. FDG-avid or PET+ before therapy: PET+ at prior sites of diseases and no new sites on CT or PET b. Variably FDG-avid or PET−: no change in size of previous lesions on CT	—	—

Relapsed or progressive disease	Any new lesion or increase by ≥50% of previously involved sites from nadir	Appearance of a new lesion >1.5 cm in any axis, ≥50% in the longest diameter of a previously identified node >1 cm in short axis or in the SPD of more than one node. Lesions PET+ if FDG-avid lymphoma or PET+ before therapy	≥50% increase from nadir in the SPD of any previous lesions	New or recurrent involvement

Data from Cheson BD, Pfistner B, Juweid ME, et al. Revised response criteria for malignant lymphoma. J Clin Oncol. 2007;25:579–86.

Stable Disease

Failing to attain the criteria needed for a CR or PR, but not fulfilling those for progressive disease (see below).

Typically FGD-avid lymphomas: the FDG-PET should be positive at prior sites of
disease with no new areas of involvement on the posttreatment CT or PET.

Variably FDG-avid lymphomas/FDG-avidity unknown: For patients who had no
pretreatment PET scan or if the pretreatment PET was negative, there must be
no change in the size of the previous lesions on the posttreatment CT scan.

Relapsed Disease (After Complete Response)/Progressive Disease (After Partial Response, Stable Disease)

Lymph nodes should be considered abnormal if the long axis is >1.5 cm regardless of the short axis. If a lymph node has a long axis of 1.1 to 1.5 cm it
should only be considered abnormal if its short axis is >1.0. Lymph nodes
≤1.0 cm × ≤1.0 cm are not considered as abnormal for relapse or progressive
disease.

Appearance of any new lesion >1.5 cm in any axis during or at the end of therapy, even if others are decreasing in size. Increased FDG uptake in a previously unaffected site should only be considered relapsed or progressive
disease after confirmation with other modalities. In patients who had no prior
history of pulmonary lymphoma, new lung nodules identified by CT are
mostly benign. A therapeutic decision should not be made solely on the basis
of the PET without histologic confirmation.

A ≥50% increase from nadir in the SPD of any previously involved nodes, or in
a single involved node, or the size of other lesions (eg, splenic or hepatic
nodules). To be considered progressive disease, a lymph node with a diameter of the short axis of <1.0 cm must increase by ≥50% and to a size of 1.5
× 1.5 cm or >1.5 cm in the long axis.

A ≥50% increase in the longest diameter of any single previously identified
node >1 cm in its short axis.

Lesions should be PET-positive if a typical FDG-avid lymphoma or one that was
PET-positive before therapy, unless the lesion is too small to be detected with
current PET systems (<1.5 cm in its long axis by CT).

Measurable extranodal disease should be assessed in a manner similar to
nodal disease. Disease that is only evaluable (eg, pleural effusions, bone lesions)
is recorded as present or absent only, unless an abnormality that is still noted
by imaging studies or physical examination is found to be histologically
negative.

For clinical trials in which PET is unavailable to the vast majority of partic-
ipants or PET is not deemed necessary or appropriate, response should be assessed as above, but only using CT scans. Residual masses should not be
assigned CRu status, however, but should be considered partial responses.

FOLLOW-UP EVALUATION

The most important components of monitoring patients following treatment
are a careful history and physical examination and good clinical judgment.

Laboratory testing at follow-up visits should include CBC and serum chemistries, including LDH and other relevant blood tests. Recently, the National Comprehensive Cancer Network published recommendations for follow-up of patients who have Hodgkin's and non-Hodgkin's lymphoma [42,43]: for patients who have Hodgkin's lymphoma in an initial complete remission, an interim history and physical examination every 2 to 4 months for 1 to 2 years, then every 3 to 6 months for the next 3 to 5 years, with annual monitoring for late effects after 5 years. Imaging studies should be performed when clinically indicated. There is no evidence to support regular surveillance CT or PET scans because the patient or physician identifies the relapse more than 80% of the time [44–48].

ENDPOINTS FOR CLINICAL TRIALS

The International Harmonization Project also standardized endpoints for clinical trials to ensure comparability among studies (Table 2). These are divided into the response-related endpoints described above (eg, CR, PR), and time-dependent endpoints. Response rates are important in phase II trials of novel new agents in which identification of clinical activity is generally a primary objective. Improved response rates do not always translate into prolonged time-dependent endpoints, especially in the incurable histologies [49]. Randomized studies provide the best determination of benefit in time-dependent variables (progression-free survival, event-free survival) because historical controls are subject to bias and therefore unreliable.

DEFINITIONS OF TIME-DEPENDENT AND OTHER ENDPOINTS

Overall Survival

Overall survival is the time from entry onto the clinical trial until death from any cause (Table 3). Although survival is unambiguous, it is not always an optimal endpoint because of the time it may take to achieve that endpoint and because it may reflect the effects of subsequent therapies.

Progression-Free Survival

Progression-free survival (PFS) is defined as the time from entry onto study until lymphoma progression or death from any cause. PFS is often the preferred endpoint in lymphoma clinical trials, especially those involving incurable or indolent histologies, because it reflects tumor growth and therefore is interpretable earlier than the endpoint of overall survival and is not confounded by subsequent therapies.

Event-Free Survival

Event-free survival (time to treatment failure) is measured from the time from study entry to any treatment failure, including disease progression or discontinuation of treatment for any reason (eg, disease progression, toxicity, patient preference, initiation of new treatment without documented progression, or death). This endpoint is generally not encouraged by regulatory agencies

Table 3
Efficacy endpoints

	Patients	Definition	Measured from
Primary endpoints			
Overall survival	All	Death from any cause	Entry onto study
Progression-free survival	All	Diseases progression or death from any cause	Entry onto study
Secondary endpoints			
Event-free survival	All	Failure of treatment or death from any cause	Entry onto study
Time to progression	All	Time to progression or death from lymphoma	Entry onto study
Disease-free survival	In CR	Time to relapse or death from lymphoma or acute toxicity of treatment	Documentation of response
Response duration	In CR or PR	Time to relapse or progression	Documentation of response
Lymphoma-specific survival	All	Time to death from lymphoma	Entry onto study
Time to next treatment	All	Time to new treatment	End of primary treatment

Data from Cheson BD, Pfistner B, Juweid ME, et al. Revised response criteria for malignant lymphoma. J Clin Oncol 2007;25:579–86.

because it is a composite of efficacy, toxicity, and patient withdrawal. It may be useful in the evaluation of some toxic therapies, however.

Time to Progression

Time to progression (TTP) is defined as the time from study entry until documented lymphoma progression or death attributable to lymphoma. In TTP, deaths from other causes are censored either at the time of death or at an earlier time of assessment, representing a random pattern of loss from the study. TTP may be useful in curable histologies, such as Hodgkin's lymphoma, in which most deaths on a study may be unrelated to the lymphoma and instead caused by toxicity of the treatment and/or prolonged follow-up.

Disease-Free Survival

Disease-free survival is measured from the time of occurrence of disease-free state or attainment of a complete remission to disease recurrence or death from lymphoma or acute toxicity of treatment. This endpoint may be complicated by deaths that occur during the follow-up period that are unrelated to the lymphoma. Whether such deaths should be considered as events or censored at the time of occurrence is controversial because it is not always possible to identify those deaths related to the lymphoma, leading to the potential for bias.

Response Duration

Response duration is from the time when criteria for response (ie, CR or PR) are met, with the event being first documentation of relapse or progression.

Lymphoma-Specific Survival

Lymphoma-specific survival (eg, disease-specific survival, cause-specific survival) is defined as time from study entry to death from lymphoma. This endpoint is potentially subject to bias because the exact cause of death is not always easy to ascertain. To minimize the risk for bias, an event should be recorded as death from lymphoma, or from toxicity from the drug. Death from unknown causes should be attributed to the therapy.

Time to Next Treatment

For certain trials, time to next lymphoma treatment may be of interest, defined as time from the end of primary treatment until the institution of the next therapy.

Clinical Benefit

Clinical benefit is one of the most important, but least well defined, endpoints in clinical trials. It may reflect an improvement in quality of life; a reduction in patient symptoms, transfusion requirements, and frequent infections; or other parameters. Time to reappearance or progression of lymphoma-related symptoms can also be used in this endpoint.

The International Harmonization Project developed these revised guidelines with the goal of improved comparability among studies, leading to accelerated new agent development resulting in the rapid availability of improved therapies for patients who have lymphoma. Modifications of these recommendations are expected as new information and improved technologies become available.

References

[1] Grillo-López AJ, Cheson BD, Horning SJ, et al. Response criteria for NHL: importance of "normal" lymph node size and correlations with response rates. Ann Oncol 2000;11: 399–408.

[2] Cheson BD, Horning SJ, Coiffier B, et al. Report of an International Workshop to standardize response criteria for non-Hodgkin's lymphomas. J Clin Oncol 1999;17:1244–53.

[3] Surbone A, Longo DL, DeVita VT Jr, et al. Residual abdominal masses in aggressive non-Hodgkin's lymphoma after combination chemotherapy: significance and management. J Clin Oncol 1988;6:1832–7.

[4] Radford JA, Cowan RA, Flanagan M, et al. The significance of residual mediastinal abnormality on the chest radiograph following treatment for Hodgkin's disease. J Clin Oncol 1988;6:940–6.

[5] Bangerter M, Moog F, Buchmann I, et al. Whole-body 2-[18F]-fluoro-2-deoxy-D-glucose positron emission tomography (FDG-PET) for accurate staging of Hodgkin's disease. Ann Oncol 1998;9:1117–22.

[6] Spaepen K, Stroobants S, Dupont P, et al. Prognostic value of positron emission tomography (PET) with fluorine-18 fluorodeoxyglucose ([18F]FDG) after first-line chemotherapy in non-Hodgkin's lymphoma: Is [18F]FDG-PET a valid alternative to conventional diagnostic methods? J Clin Oncol 2001;19:414–9.

[7] Spaepen K, Stroobants S, Dupont P, et al. Prognostic value of pretransplantation positron emission tomography using fluorine 18-fluorodeoxyglucose in patients with aggressive lymphoma treated with high-dose chemotherapy and stem cell transplantation. Blood 2003;102:53–9.

[8] Spaepen K, Stroobants S, Dupont P, et al. Early restaging positron emission tomography with 18F-fluorodeoxyglucose predicts outcome in patients with aggressive non-Hodgkin's lymphoma. Ann Oncol 2002;13:1356–63.

[9] Jerusalem G, Beguin Y, Fassotte MF, et al. Whole-body positron emission tomography using 18F-fluorodeoxyglucose compared to standard procedures for staging patients with Hodgkin's disease. Haematologica 2001;86:266–73.

[10] Jerusalem G, Beguin Y, Fassotte MF, et al. Whole-body positron emission tomography using 18F-fluorodeoxyglucose for posttreatment evaluation in Hodgkin's disease and non-Hodgkin's lymphoma has higher diagnostic and prognostic value than classical computed tomography scan imaging. Blood 1999;94:429–33.

[11] Jerusalem G, Beguin Y, Najjar F, et al. Positron emission tomography (PET) with 18F-fluorodeoxyglucose (18F-FDG) for the staging of low-grade non-Hodgkin's lymphoma (NHL). Ann Oncol 2001;12:825–30.

[12] Jerusalem G, Warland V, Najjar F, et al. Whole-body 18F-FDG PET for the evaluation of patients with Hodgkin's disease and non-Hodgkin's lymphoma. Nucl Med Commun 1999;20: 13–20.

[13] Zinzani PL, Magagnoli M, Chierichetti F, et al. The role of positron emission tomography (PET) in the management of lymphoma patients. Ann Oncol 1999;10:1141–3.

[14] Weihrauch MR, Re D, Scheidhauer K, et al. Thoracic positron emission tomography using 18F-fluorodeoxyglucose for the evaluation of residual mediastinal Hodgkin disease. Blood 2001;98:2930–4.

[15] Naumann R, Vaic A, Beuthien-Baumann B, et al. Prognostic value of positron emission tomography in the evaluation of post-treatment residual mass in patients with Hodgkin's disease and non-Hodgkin's lymphoma. Br J Haematol 2001;115:793–800.

[16] Kostakoglu L, Leonard JP, Kuji I, et al. Comparison of fluorine-18 fluorodeoxyglucose positron emission tomography and Ga-67 scintigraphy in evaluation of lymphoma. Cancer 2002;94:879–88.

[17] Naumann R, Beuthien-Baumann B, Reiss A, et al. Substantial impact of FDG PET imaging on the therapy decision in patients with early-stage Hodgkin's lymphoma. Br J Cancer 2004;90:620–5.

[18] Munker R, Glass J, Griffeth LK, et al. Contribution of PET imaging to the initial staging and prognosis of patients with Hodgkin's disease. Ann Oncol 2004;15:1699–704.

[19] Mikhaeel NG, Hutchings M, Fields PA, et al. FDG-PET after two to three cycles of chemotherapy predicts progression-free and overall survival in high-grade non-Hodgkin lymphoma. Ann Oncol 2005;16:1514–23.

[20] Juweid M, Cheson BD. Positron emission tomography (PET) in post-therapy assessment of cancer. N Engl J Med 2005;354:496–507.

[21] Juweid M, Wiseman GA, Vose JM, et al. Response assessment of aggressive non-Hodgkin's lymphoma by integrated International Workshop criteria (IWC) and 18F-fluorodeoxyglucose positron emission tomography (PET). J Clin Oncol 2005;23: 4652–61.

[22] Haioun C, Itti E, Rahmouni A, et al. [18F]fluoro-2-deoxy-D-glucose positron emission tomography (FDG-PET) in aggressive lymphoma: an early prognostic tool for predicting patient outcome. Blood 2005;106:1376–81.

[23] Hutchings M, Loft A, Hansen M, et al. Positron emission tomography with or without computed tomography in the primary staging of Hodgkin's lymphoma. Haematologica 2006;91:482–9.

[24] Querellou S, Valette F, Bodet-Milin C, et al. FDG-PET/CT predicts outcome in patients with aggressive non-Hodgkin's lymphoma and Hodgkin's disease. Ann Hematol 2006;85: 759–67.

[25] Gallamini A, Rigacci L, Merli F, et al. Predictive value of positron emission tomography performed after two courses of standard therapy on treatment outcome in advanced stage Hodgkin's disease. Haematologica 2006;91:475–81.

[26] Hutchings M, Loft A, Hansen M, et al. FDG-PET after two cycles of chemotherapy predicts treatment failure and progression-free survival in Hodgkin lymphoma. Blood 2006;107: 52–9.

[27] Juweid ME, Stroobants S, Hoekstra OS, et al. Use of positron emission tomography for response assessment of lymphoma: consensus recommendations of the Imaging Subcommittee of the International Harmonization Project in Lymphoma. J Clin Oncol 2007;25: 571–8.

[28] Cheson BD, Pfistner B, Juweid ME, et al. Revised response criteria for malignant lymphoma. J Clin Oncol 2007;25:579–86.

[29] Buchmann I, Reinhardt M, Elsner K, et al. 2-(fluorine-18)fluoro-2-deoxy-D-glucose positron emission tomography in the detection and staging of malignant lymphoma. A bicenter trial. Cancer 2001;91:889–99.

[30] Stumpe KD, Urbinelli M, Steinert HC, et al. Whole-body positron emission tomography using fluorodeoxyglucose for staging of lymphoma: effectiveness and comparison with computed tomography. Eur J Nucl Med 1998;25:721–8.

[31] Wirth A, Seymour JF, Hicks RJ, et al. Fluorine-18 fluorodeoxyglucose positron emission tomography, gallium-67 scintigraphy, and conventional staging for Hodgkin's disease and non-Hodgkin's lymphoma. Am J Med 2002;112:262–8.

[32] Hoffmann M, Kletter K, Diemling M, et al. Positron emission tomography with fluorine-18-2-fluoro-2-deoxy-D-glucose (F18-FDG) does not visualize extranodal B-cell lymphoma of the mucosa-associated lymphoid tissue (MALT)-type. Ann Oncol 1999;10:1185–9.

[33] Elstrom R, Guan L, Baker G, et al. Utility of FDG-PET scanning in lymphoma by WHO classification. Blood 2003;101:3875–6.

[34] Karam M, Novak L, Cyriac J, et al. Role of fluorine-18 fluoro-deoxyglucose positron emission tomography scan in the evaluation and follow-up of patients with low-grade lymphomas. Cancer 2006;107:175–83.

[35] Hoffmann M, Wöhrer S, Becherer A, et al. 18F-fluoro-deoxy-glucose positron emission tomography in lymphoma of mucosa-associated lymphoid tissue: histology makes the difference. Ann Oncol 2006;17:1761–5.

[36] Lewis PJ, Salama A. Uptake of fluorine-18-flouorodeoxyglucose in sarcoidosis. J Nucl Med 1994;35:1647–9.

[37] Castellucci P, Nanni C, Farsad M, et al. Potential pitfalls of ^{18}F-FDG PET in a large series of patients treated for malignant lymphoma: prevalence and scan interpretation. Nucl Med Commun 2005;26:689–94.

[38] Pfistner B, Diehl V, Cheson B. International harmonization of trial parameters in malignant lymphoma. Eur J Haematol Suppl 2005;(66):53–4.

[39] Kostakoglu L, Coleman M, Leonard JP, et al. PET predicts prognosis after 1 cycle of chemotherapy in aggressive lymphoma and Hodgkin's disease. J Nucl Med 2002;43: 1018–27.

[40] Zinzani PL, Tani M, Fanti S, et al. Early positron emission tomography (PET) restaging: a predictive final response in Hodgkin's disease patients. Ann Oncol 2006;17:1296–300.

[41] Kelloff GJ, Krohn KA, Larson SM, et al. The progress and promise of molecular imaging probes in oncologic drug development. Clin Cancer Res 2005;15:7967–85.

[42] Hoppe RT, Advani RH, Bierman PJ, et al. Hodgkin disease/lymphoma. Clinical practice guidelines in oncology. J Natl Compr Canc Netw 2006;4(3):210–30.

[43] Zelenetz AD, Advani RH, Buadi F, et al. Non-Hodgkin's lymphoma: clinical practice guidelines in oncology. J Natl Compr Canc Netw 2006;4(3):258–310.

[44] Weeks JC, Yeap BY, Canellos GP, et al. Value of follow-up procedures in patients with large-cell lymphoma who achieve a complete remission. J Clin Oncol 1991;9:1196–203.

[45] Oh YK, Ha CS, Samuels BI, et al. Stages I–III follicular lymphoma: role of CT of the abdomen and pelvis in follow-up studies. Radiology 1999;210:483–6.

[46] Foltz LM, Song KW, Connors JM. Who actually detects relapse in Hodgkin lymphoma: patient or physician? [abstract 3124]. Blood 2004;104(part 1):853a–4a.

[47] Liedtke M, Hamlin PA, Moskowitz CH, et al. Surveillance imaging during remission identifies a group of patients with more favorable aggressive NHL at time of relapse: a retrospective analysis of a uniformly-treated patient population. Ann Oncol 2006;17:909–13.

[48] Jerusalem G, Beguin Y, Fassotte MF, et al. Early detection of relapse by whole-body positron emission tomography in the follow-up of patients with Hodgkin's disease. Ann Oncol 2003;14:123–30.

[49] Kimby E, Björkholm M, Gahrton G, et al. Chlorambucil/prednisone vs. CHOP in symptomatic low-grade non-Hodgkin's lymphomas: a randomized trial from the Lymphoma Group of Central Sweden. Ann Oncol 1994;5(Suppl 2):67–71.

Is [18F]fluorodeoxyglucose Positron Emission Tomography the Ultimate Tool for Response and Prognosis Assessment?

Lieselot Brepoels, MD*, Sigrid Stroobants, MD, PhD

Division of Nuclear Medicine, University Hospital Gasthuisberg, Herestraat 49,
B-3000 Leuven, Belgium

Combined chemo- and radiotherapy have increased the cure rate for Hodgkin's lymphoma (HL) to more than 80% to 90%. A major concern has been the late toxic effects of treatment, however, most of which are attributable to consolidation radiotherapy. Patients who received mediastinal radiotherapy have an increased risk of fatal myocardial infarction [1], heart valve fibrosis [2], restrictive cardiomyopathy, and conduction abnormalities [3]. The approximately 3% lifetime risk of acute leukemia has long been recognized [4] and the risk of second malignancies is 22% to 27% at 25 to 30 years following treatment for HL [5–9]. In early-stage HL, treatment-related illness accounts for more deaths than HL itself [10].

The ultimate goal is therefore to minimize these side effects without losing treatment efficacy. This understanding has questioned the standard use of radiotherapy in early-stage HL and urges us to tailor the intensity of the treatment to the individual patient (reduce if possible, intensify if needed). Risk-adapted strategies require early and accurate assessment of response, which traditionally is done by CT. Response evaluation by CT imaging does not allow identification of patients who will benefit from consolidation radiotherapy and those who will not, however. This fact has recently been illustrated by the preliminary results of the collaboration between the European Organisation for Research and Treatment of Cancer and Le Groupe d'Etudes des Lymphomes de L'Adulte (EORTC-GELA) H9-F trial, in which patients who had favorable-stage HL who obtained complete remission (CR) or unconfirmed complete remission (CRu) on CT imaging, were randomized between no radiotherapy and low- or high-dose radiotherapy. Inclusion of patients in the no-radiotherapy arm had to be stopped prematurely because of an unacceptable high failure

Lieselot Brepoels is a Research Assistant of the Flemish Fund for Scientific Research (FWO Vlaanderen).

*Corresponding author. E-mail address: lieselot.brepoels@uz.kuleuven.be (L. Brepoels).

0889-8588/07/$ – see front matter
doi:10.1016/j.hoc.2007.07.003
© 2007 Elsevier Inc. All rights reserved.
hemonc.theclinics.com

rate (69% event-free survival versus 85% and 89% in low- and high-dose radio-therapy group) [11]. Clearly, a more accurate tool to select patients who have a good prognosis in whom additional radiotherapy can be omitted is needed; positron emission tomography (PET) using the radiolabeled glucose analog [18F]fluorodeoxyglucose (FDG) may be useful in this setting.

[18F]FLUORODEOXYGLUCOSE POSITRON EMISSION TOMOGRAPHY FOR RESPONSE EVALUATION AT THE END OF THERAPY

Literature Data

Numerous studies have shown the effectiveness of FDG-PET in the detection of residual HL at the end of therapy and the more accurate assessment of the remission status compared with CT [12–21]. A high negative predictive value (NPV) of 81% to 100% is consistently reported in most studies, and PET clearly identifies patients who have an excellent prognosis. In a recent systematic review, Zijlstra and colleagues [22] pooled the results of 15 studies evaluating PET after first-line treatment in lymphoma. Subgroup analysis in 247 patients who had HL showed a sensitivity and specificity of 84% and 90% for the detection of residual lymphoma. Relapses in PET-negative patients are infrequent and occur rarely within the first year after the end of treatment, probably reflecting minimal tumor burden below the detection limit of the PET system at the time of restaging. Because a substantial number of patients received additional radiotherapy after a negative PET scan, however, reported NPV may be overestimated. The question whether radiotherapy can be omitted in early-stage HL with a negative PET scan after first-line chemotherapy is therefore still unanswered. Furthermore, almost all patients who have early-stage HL have a negative end-of-treatment PET and survive without relapse, reflecting probably more the excellent prognosis of these patients than the high sensitivity of PET.

An important but less consistent feature of PET response evaluation in HL is the incidence of false-positive lesions (reported positive predictive value between 25% and 100%), especially in studies focusing on patients who have residual masses (Table 1). The finding of nontumoral, false-positive FDG uptake is not infrequent and was described by Castellucci and colleagues [23] in about 3% of 1000 PET scans in patients who had suspected relapse of lymphoma. This incidence makes it mandatory to confirm suspected results on PET by histology or other imaging modalities before starting additional or salvage treatment (Fig. 1).

False-Positive Lesions on [18F]fluorodeoxyglucose Positron Emission Tomography for Response Evaluation at the End of Therapy

False-positive FDG uptake inside a residual mass, although rare, is more frequent after radiation therapy or chemoradiation than after chemotherapy alone and is caused by transient inflammatory changes as a reaction to therapy. It is therefore recommended to wait at least 3, and preferably 6 to 8, weeks after

Table 1
Predictive value of end-of-treatment positron emission tomography in a population of Hodgkin's lymphoma

Author	Number of patients	PPV (%)	NPV (%)	Accuracy (%)	Median follow-up (mo)
Lavely et al, [12]	20	ns	81	ns	36
Weihrauch et al, [13]	28	60	84	76	28
Panizo et al, [14]	29	75	100	90	28
Friedberg et al, [15]	32	50	96	84	24
Jerusalem et al, [16]	36	100	94	83	>36
de Wit et al, [17]	37	46	96	74	26
Naumann et al, [18]	43	25	100	93	35
Heultenschmidt et al, [19]	47	86	96	91	20
Guay et al, [20]	48	92	92	92	16
Spaepen et al, [21]	60	100	91	92	32

Abbreviations: NPV, negative predictive value; ns, not specified; PPV, positive predictive value.

chemotherapy or chemoimmunotherapy, and 8 to 12 weeks after radiation or chemoradiation [24]. This FDG uptake inside a residual mass is typically marked by a diffuse, slightly increased uptake that tends to decrease over time. Because of this typical finding, some authors created a category of "minimal residual uptake" (MRU) on PET in addition to the classification of a positive or negative PET. This MRU interpretation is rather vague, differs between studies, is largely observer-dependent, and the obtained results in these patients are open for extensive discussions [25]. To overcome this

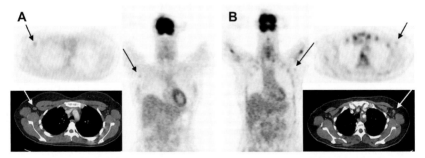

Fig. 1. PET and CT images in two patients who were treated for HL and presented with residual FDG uptake in a slightly enlarged lymph node. Patient A had active erysipelas at the right thumb at the time of PET evaluation, and because an inflammatory lymph node was suspected no additional treatment was given. The patient remains in remission after a follow-up of 36 months. Residual FDG uptake in patient B was caused by persistent lymphoma and he relapsed in the left axilla after a follow-up of 4 months.

indistinctness in classification, a comparison between FDG uptake in the residual mass and the mediastinal blood pool structures has been proposed as a reference cutoff for standardization of PET results [24,26]. Residual masses larger than 2 cm, with uptake lower than or equal to mediastinal blood pool structures, should be considered negative for lymphoma, whereas uptake exceeding that of the mediastinum is suggestive of residual disease. Because FDG uptake in a small residual mass (<2 cm) is artificially decreased because of the low resolution of PET systems, any uptake higher than local background should be considered positive for residual lymphoma in these small lesions (see the article by Cheson and colleagues in this issue). Whether this guideline will indeed lead to a decrease in false-positive results is still to be confirmed.

False-positive lesions outside a previously involved area can be caused by physiologic FDG uptake in muscles, brown fat, gut, and the urinary excretion system. False-positive FDG uptake can also be seen in contemporaneous pathology as inflammation and other malignant or benign tumors (eg, thyroid adenoma). In younger patients, diffuse butterfly-shaped uptake in the anterior mediastinum is mostly attributable to thymus hyperplasia. Close correlation of PET results with other imaging modalities and clinical history is therefore always mandatory. Both Reske [27] and Spaepen and colleagues [28] stated the value of a pretreatment scan for reducing false-positive PET results by allowing comparison with the posttreatment scan. The importance of performing pretreatment PET has decreased with present evolution to integrated PET/CT systems, however, because false-positive lesions can often be recognized by correlation with the CT images. Since the introduction of combined PET/CT systems, specificity and sensitivity and reader confidence have increased compared with PET alone, CT alone, or the visual correlation of PET and CT, and these integrated systems rapidly became standard in most countries [29–31].

False Negative Lesions by [^{18}F]fluorodeoxyglucose Positron Emission Tomography for Response Evaluation at the End of Therapy

Despite its high sensitivity, a completely negative PET scan cannot exclude minimal residual disease and some patients will relapse regardless of a completely negative posttreatment PET. Especially in regions with high background activity, as for example the brain, small amounts of residual lymphoma may be missed. The role of FDG-PET in the evaluation of meningeal or cerebral involvement by HL therefore remains unclear [32].

Another point of controversy is the ability of PET to evaluate bone marrow infiltration in lymphoma. Diffuse bone marrow involvement without focal bone lesions is frequently false negative on PET and cannot be differentiated from reactive bone marrow as is often seen after the administration of chemotherapy and in young patients who have newly diagnosed HL. A recent meta-analysis performed by Pakos and colleagues [33] in a mixed population of newly diagnosed HL and non-Hodgkin's lymphoma (NHL) showed that only about half of the patients who had bone marrow infiltration detected in bone marrow biopsy (BMB) were also suspect by FDG-PET. On the other hand, focal bone lesions on FDG-PET in the presence of negative BMB often indicate missed bone marrow involvement because of sampling error, which can be documented with a second BMB directed at the site of a positive PET signal. The techniques are therefore considered complementary.

An analogous pattern is recognized in organ involvement by lymphoma, as for example in spleen and liver involvement. Although PET is highly sensitive for multifocal organ involvement, diffuse involvement by lymphoma may be missed. To define diffuse involvement by lymphoma in the spleen, comparison with FDG uptake in the (normal) liver is proposed as a guideline, and uptake exceeding liver uptake is considered suggestive for lymphoma (Fig. 2) [24]. Although the value of PET in detecting diffuse organ involvement is limited, the sensitivity of conventional imaging techniques for the detection is even worse, and FDG-PET is therefore considered the more accurate tool for the response evaluation in case of diffuse organ involvement.

In contrast to diffuse lymphoma involvement, PET is considered highly specific and sensitive for the detection of focal lesions in the spleen or liver. Focal lesions after therapy that are 1.5 cm or larger on CT are considered negative for lymphoma if their uptake is lower than that of the surrounding liver or spleen. For lesions less than 1.5 cm, uptake equal to the liver is also considered negative because the low resolution of PET limits the detection of cold lesions in a high background region [24,26].

Conclusion

Owing to its high sensitivity and specificity, FDG-PET is the imaging technique of choice for the end-of-treatment evaluation in patients who have HL.

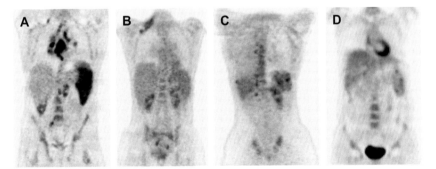

Fig. 2. Diffusely (A, B) and focally (C, D) increased FDG uptake in the spleen in patients who had Hodgkin's lymphoma (HL). Patient A is a classic example of diffusely increased FDG uptake in an enlarged spleen. Patient B presented with a normal-sized spleen with only slightly increased FDG uptake compared with liver uptake. Both patients had diffuse splenic involvement by HL. Focal lesions in the spleen were seen in patient C, which were caused by HL, and although patient D was initially believed to have residual disease in the spleen based on a heterogeneous uptake, microscopic examination showed only arguments for extramedullary hematopoiesis.

Suspected abnormalities on PET should be confirmed by biopsy or other imaging modalities before starting additional or salvage treatment.

The question remains whether radiotherapy may be omitted based on end-of-treatment PET in an individual patient and several initiatives have recently been started to answer this question.

PROGNOSTIC VALUE OF EARLY RESPONSE ASSESSMENT BY [¹⁸F]FLUORODEOXYGLUCOSE POSITRON EMISSION TOMOGRAPHY

The most frequently used chemotherapy regimen for HL is ABVD (Adriamycin, bleomycin, vincristine, dexamethasone), which was introduced in the 1970s. The German Hodgkin's Study Group (GHSG) has shown a superior remission rate with a more intensive regimen (BEACOPP) in patients who have advanced disease [34]. Because patients who have poor prognoses may benefit from these upfront intensified treatment regimens, it is useful to know the individual patient's risk for relapse as early as possible. Pretreatment prognostic indicators, such as disease stage, number of involved regions, B symptoms, extranodal and bulky disease, age, and biochemical parameters, have been shown to predict survival in large cohort studies. Investigators and clinicians often use combinations of these factors at diagnosis to define subgroups of patients who have high or low risk of relapse and to identify those patients who would benefit from intensified strategies and those who could be cured with less toxic treatments. Among others, the most frequently used prognostic model in HL is the International Prognostic Score (IPS) [35]. The use of these scoring systems is controversial, however, because they show low efficacy and a limited predictive power [36]. The upfront use of risk-adapted therapy based on these models is even more controversial as a significant increase in long-term side effects is expected in patients who have a substantial chance to be cured with less toxic treatment regimens. Conversely, a substantial proportion of patients who are falsely stratified in the low-risk category may be under-treated.

Probably more important than the extent of disease at diagnosis is the individual sensitivity of the tumor to the initially installed treatment. Despite the overall high cure rate in HL, some patients fail to reach remission after first-line therapy and these nonresponders have a much worse prognosis. They need to be identified as early as possible to avoid treatment failure and needless toxicity. Conventional imaging techniques, such as CT, are not very useful to differentiate responders from nonresponders early during treatment because tumor shrinkage takes time and therefore anatomic changes only appear after several cycles of chemotherapy (Fig. 3). Metabolic changes precede the anatomic ones, however, and within a few days after the administration of a chemotherapeutic agent, a reduction in number and metabolism of the viable lymphoma cells can be seen [37]. Because FDG uptake is closely related to the metabolic activity and the number of viable cells, effective treatment results in a fast reduction of the FDG uptake, making PET a sensitive and early marker of response. The rationale for

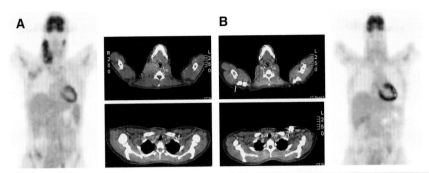

Fig. 3. Pre- (A) and mid-treatment (B) PET and CT in a patient who had HL in the cervical region. Mid-treatment CT shows residual enlarged lymph nodes without residual increased FDG uptake on PET. The patient remains in CR after a follow-up of 24 months.

performing PET early during therapy lies in the detection of resistant clones that respond to treatment more slowly than chemosensitive tumor cells and may eventually cause disease relapse or progression.

Römer [38] was the first to document a rapid decrease of FDG uptake as early as 7 days after treatment in 11 patients who had NHL. Based on these findings, several authors have investigated the use of PET for response assessment early during the course of chemotherapy (Table 2). Mikhaeel and colleagues [39] was the first to report on the value of early PET in a population of exclusively HL. In this study involving 32 patients, PET response assessment was performed after two to three cycles of chemotherapy. All 6 patients who had persistent abnormalities on PET relapsed compared with only 2 of 26 (8%) complete responders. Hutchings and colleagues [40] prospectively compared FDG-PET after two and four cycles of therapy and at the end of treatment in 77 patients who had HL. A positive PET after two cycles of therapy was highly predictive for progression with a 2-year progression free survival (PFS) of 0% compared with 96% for PET-negative patients. PET after two cycles was as accurate as after four cycles and at the end of treatment, and superior to CT at all time points. Gallamini and colleagues [41] confirmed these results in 108 patients who had advanced-stage HL or adverse prognostic factors, and showed a 2-year disease-free survival of 6% in PET-positive and 96% in PET-negative patients. In both studies, early FDG-PET proved to be an independent prognostic factor with a predictive value higher than any of the other prognostic factors.

In a clinical situation, it is important to know as soon as possible whether a treatment will be effective. Kostakoglu and colleagues [42] looked at the value of PET after 1 month of therapy in newly diagnosed diffuse large cell lymphoma (DLCL, n = 24) and HL (n = 23). All 31 PET-negative patients had sustained complete remission with a median follow-up of 28 months, and 14 of 16 PET-positive patients had refractory disease or relapsed. Of these last 16 PET-positive patients, 4 patients were converted to negative on

Table 2
Prognostic value of positron emission tomography for early response assessment during first-line or induction treatment (selection of the studies mentioned in the text)

Author	No. of patients	Histology	Timing PET (cycles)	Sensitivity (%)	Specificity (%)	Accuracy (%)	PPV (%)	NPV (%)	Follow-up (mo)
Mikhaeel et al, [39]	32	HL	2-3	75	100	94	100	92	36
Friedberg et al, [15]	22	HL	3	80	94	91	80	94	24
Hutchings et al, [40]	77	HL	2	79	92	90	69	95	23
	64	HL	4	85	96	94	85	96	23
Gallamini et al, [41]	108	HL	2	86	98	95	90	97	20
Römer et al, [38]	11	NHL	1	no difference in SUV between nonresponders and responders					16
	11	NHL	2	80	100	91	100	86	16
Torizuka et al, [43]	20	HL/NHL	1-2	87	50	80	87	50	24
Kostakoglu et al, [42]	47	HL/DLCL	1	100	94	96	88	100	28

Abbreviations: DLCL, diffuse large cell lymphoma; HL, Hodgkin's lymphoma; NHL, non-Hodgkin's lymphoma; NPV, negative predictive value; PPV, positive predictive value; SUV, standardized uptake value.

end-of-treatment PET but 3 of those 4 patients relapsed during follow-up (2 DLCL, 1 HL), which suggested a higher predictive value of PET after 1 month compared with end-of-treatment PET.

PET response is usually defined as an (almost) complete normalization of the FDG uptake and can easily be assessed visually. Although this occurs early after the start of treatment, assessment of response even earlier (eg, a few days after initiation of therapy), probably requires quantification of FDG uptake and the use of threshold values (percentage decrease from baseline or amount of residual FDG uptake). In the study by Römer and colleagues [38], four of six responders had significant residual FDG uptake 1 week after the start of treatment.

Quantification on FDG-PET is usually expressed by standardized uptake value (SUV), which is a measurement for FDG uptake at a certain location in the body, normalized to the injected dose of FDG. Torizuka and colleagues [43] quantitatively investigated the decrease in SUV in a population of 20 lymphoma patients (17 NHL, 3 HL) and found that tumor SUVs after one to two cycles of therapy were significantly lower in the group of responders compared with the group of nonresponders. Using 60% reduction in SUV as a cutoff value, the group of responders could be clearly separated from the group of nonresponders, with the exception of one nonresponder. Hutchings and colleagues [40] showed a cutoff value of 4 for the maximal SUV (SUV_{max}) as the optimal balancing point between sensitivity and specificity for PET after two cycles of chemotherapy. Furthermore, receiver operating characteristic tables in this study showed 100% specificity for SUV_{max} greater than 5 and 100% sensitivity for SUV_{max} less than 3. In the study by Kostakoglu and colleagues [42], the optimal cutoff was 1.75 for the average SUV_{max} after one cycle of chemotherapy. By using this SUV_{max} cutoff point, the sensitivity was 91.7% and the specificity was 83.7%. In each of these studies, however, cutoff values were determined by the distribution of SUVs in their own population and are therefore not necessarily reproducible in a different patient group. Moreover, it is not unlikely that rapidity of FDG response differs between treatment modalities and types of drugs, so that cutoff values and timing of PET scanning should be adapted to the treatment strategy used.

Risk-Adapted Treatment Modifications Based on Early [^{18}F]fluorodeoxyglucose Positron Emission Tomography

Dann and colleagues [44] was the first to demonstrate that risk-adapted treatment in HL can reduce the cumulative dose of chemotherapy without impairment of outcome. Patients who have newly diagnosed HL and adverse prognostic factors were assigned to their initial regimen (standard or escalated BEACOPP) based on the IPS, and the therapy was adjusted based on the response by FDG-PET/ CT scanning after two cycles. Following a negative interim scan, four cycles of standard BEACOPP were administered, whereas four cycles of escalated BEACOPP were given to patients who had a positive scan followed by radiation therapy to the sites of FDG-uptake at the end of therapy. Among the 39 high-risk patients, treatment was decreased to standard BEACOPP in 31 patients (79%)

without reduction in 5-year event-free and overall survival. These results suggest that risk-adapted treatment, by means of IPS for initial chemotherapy and response to chemotherapy by early interim PET, may be used to decrease the dose of chemotherapy without affecting efficacy. Their study suffers, however, from the absence of a control group in which treatment remained unchanged regardless of results on early interim PET.

No other published reports have demonstrated that PET-adapted therapy improves outcome or treatment toxicity. Because clinicians in most centers tend to start salvage treatment in HL when there is evidence of persistent lymphoma at the end-of-treatment evaluation, and because early PET after a few cycles of chemotherapy adequately predicts outcome at the end of treatment, we may ask whether it is still acceptable to administer chemotherapy when it is unlikely to lead to a complete remission. Coleman and colleagues showed in 1998 that prolongation of chemotherapy did not improve response or survival in HL, which suggests that patients who are apt to respond do so during the first three to six cycles of chemotherapy [45]. Large prospective two-arm studies are currently ongoing to compare clinical outcome in patients who have a positive interim FDG-PET who either continue to receive the installed induction therapy or change to a more aggressive or more experimental treatment (EORTC-H10 trial and the GHSG-HD15 trial).

Conclusion

FDG-PET after a few cycles of chemotherapy is an important prognostic factor in HL. The negative predictive value of early interim PET is extremely high in patients who have early-stage disease, which is not surprising because early-stage HL has an excellent prognosis. Likewise, the positive predictive value is very high in advanced-stage patients. Moreover, most authors are convinced that early PET has a stronger prognostic value than end-of-treatment PET. The explanation of these superior results is probably that the rapidity of achieving a complete remission is related to a higher chemosensitivity of the tumor [46]. Whether response-adapted treatment strategies based on FDG-PET may also improve patient outcome remains to be proved.

PROGNOSTIC VALUE OF [¹⁸F]FLUORODEOXYGLUCOSE POSITRON EMISSION TOMOGRAPHY IN THE PRETRANSPLANT SETTING

Patients who have a relapse of HL may benefit from intensive chemotherapy followed by myeloablative therapy and autologous stem cell support (ASCT). This treatment will only be successful in patients who still have chemosensitive disease [47]. During the last decade, FDG-PET has shown the ability to assess lymphoma activity and a positive PET before transplantation is highly predictive of early relapse with a positive predictive value ranging between 86% and 100% [48–52]. Because inflammatory disease is frequently seen in this population, correlation of PET with clinical and morphologic imaging data is essential.

Schot and colleagues [53] recently showed that the combination of clinical risk scores with PET after two courses of induction treatment provides an accurate prognostic instrument for the outcome of second-line treatment in relapsed HL and aggressive NHL. The same author also performed PET after two cycles of induction chemotherapy and after a third cycle just before ASCT to define the optimal time point for pretransplantation PET [54]. Patients who had a negative PET after the second and third cycle of chemotherapy had a 2-year PFS of 71% and 58%, respectively, whereas those who showed persistent uptake all relapsed shortly after ASCT. These results indicate that PET after three cycles had a better predictive value than PET after two cycles to identify patients who had a poor prognosis, and that patients who were positive after the second cycle still had a chance of obtaining a disease-free status after the third cycle. At the same time, PFS was longer in patients who obtained CR after the second compared with after the third cycle, which supports the hypothesis that an early response is correlated with a longer PFS.

Before PET can be used as a standard practice to determine patient eligibility for high-dose therapy with ASCT, further studies are necessary to define the optimal timing of PET and the criteria for response assessment.

POSITRON EMISSION TOMOGRAPHY FOR POSTTHERAPY SURVEILLANCE

To our knowledge only one study, by Jerusalem and colleagues [16], investigated the value of PET for the detection of preclinical relapse in 36 patients who had HL. After the end of treatment, follow-up PET was performed every 4 to 6 months for 2 to 3 years and when an abnormal FDG uptake was seen a confirmatory scan was performed 4 to 6 weeks later. In total, 11 of 36 patients had a positive scan, of whom only 5 were identified as relapse. All 5 relapses were first identified by PET before clinical examination, laboratory findings, or CT became positive. False-positive lesions were seen in six PET scans and in each case the confirmatory PET scan was normal. No relapses were seen in patients who were PET-negative.

This study illustrates that, particularly in favorable-stage HL, the risk for false-positive results is substantial compared with the low risk of relapse, which may lead to an increase in (useless) additional investigations. Moreover, even if PET can detect a high proportion of preclinical relapses, it will only be useful if this also improves survival by an earlier start of salvage therapy. The role of PET for posttherapy surveillance is controversial and large prospective studies are needed to determine whether PET is useful in this indication or not.

SUMMARY
Is FDG-PET the Ultimate Tool for Response and Prognosis Assessment?
The achievement of a complete remission is the primary objective of treatment in patients who have HL. FDG-PET is at the moment considered the most accurate and reliable tool for the assessment of response and prognosis.

PET is the most sensitive and specific technique for end-of-treatment evaluation and superior to conventional imaging techniques, especially in patients who have residual masses. Nevertheless, biopsy is always recommended to confirm a positive result on PET, before any substantial treatment alteration is made or salvage therapy is started.

Early after the initiation of therapy, FDG-PET has a high predictive value and can more accurately predict outcome than classic risk evaluation by pretreatment prognostic score systems. Whether risk-adapted treatment strategies may also improve patients outcome remains to be proved.

References

[1] Hancock SL, Tucker MA, Hoppe RT. Factors affecting late mortality from heart disease after treatment of Hodgkin's disease. JAMA 1993;270:1949–55.

[2] Hull MC, Morris CG, Pepine CJ, et al. Valvular dysfunction and carotid, subclavian, and coronary artery disease in survivors of Hodgkin lymphoma treated with radiation therapy. JAMA 2003;290:2831–7.

[3] Adams MJ, Lipsitz SR, Colan SD, et al. Cardiovascular status in long-term survivors of Hodgkin's disease treated with chest radiotherapy. J Clin Oncol 2004;22:3139–48.

[4] Blayney DW, Longo DL, Young RC, et al. Decreasing risk of leukemia with prolonged follow-up after chemotherapy and radiotherapy for Hodgkin's disease. N Engl J Med 1987;316:710–4.

[5] van Leeuwen FE, Klokman WJ, Veer MB, et al. Long-term risk of second malignancy in survivors of Hodgkin's disease treated during adolescence or young adulthood. J Clin Oncol 2000;18:487–97.

[6] Swerdlow AJ, Barber JA, Hudson GV, et al. Risk of second malignancy after Hodgkin's disease in a collaborative British cohort: the relation to age at treatment. J Clin Oncol 2000;18: 498–509.

[7] Dores GM, Metayer C, Curtis RE, et al. Second malignant neoplasms among long-term survivors of Hodgkin's disease: a population-based evaluation over 25 years. J Clin Oncol 2002;20:3484–94.

[8] Green DM, Hyland A, Barcos MP, et al. Second malignant neoplasms after treatment for Hodgkin's disease in childhood or adolescence. J Clin Oncol 2000;18:1492–9.

[9] Bhatia S, Yasui Y, Robison LL, et al. High risk of subsequent neoplasms continues with extended follow-up of childhood Hodgkin's disease: report from the Late Effects Study Group. J Clin Oncol 2003;21:4386–94.

[10] Meyer RM, Gospodarowicz MK, Connors JM, et al. Randomized comparison of ABVD chemotherapy with a strategy that includes radiation therapy in patients with limited-stage Hodgkin's lymphoma: National Cancer Institute of Canada Clinical Trials Group and the Eastern Cooperative Oncology Group. J Clin Oncol 2005;23(21):4634–42.

[11] Eghbali H, Brice P, Creemers GY, et al. Comparison of three radiation dose levels after EBVP regimen in favorable supradiaphragmatic clinical stages (CS) I-II Hodgkin's lymphoma (HL): preliminary results of the EORTC-GELA H9-F trial. American Society of Hematology (ASH) Annual Meeting [abstract 814]. Blood 2005;106.

[12] Lavely WC, Delbeke D, Greer JP, et al. FDG PET in the follow-up management of patients with newly diagnosed Hodgkin and non-Hodgkin lymphoma after first-line chemotherapy. Int J Radiat Oncol Biol Phys 2003;57(2):307–15.

[13] Weihrauch MR, Re D, Scheidhauer K, et al. Thoracic positron emission tomography using 18F-fluorodeoxyglucose for the evaluation of residual mediastinal Hodgkin disease. Blood 2001;98(10):2930–4.

[14] Panizo C, Perez-Salazar M, Bendandi M, et al. Positron emission tomography using 18F-fluorodeoxyglucose for the evaluation of residual Hodgkin's disease mediastinal masses. Leuk Lymphoma 2004;45(9):1829–33.

[15] Friedberg JW, Fischman A, Neuberg D, et al. FDG-PET is superior to gallium scintigraphy in staging and more sensitive in the follow-up of patients with de novo Hodgkin lymphoma: a blinded comparison. Leuk Lymphoma 2004;45(1):85–92.

[16] Jerusalem G, Beguin Y, Fassotte MF, et al. Early detection of relapse by whole-body positron emission tomography in the follow-up of patients with Hodgkin's disease. Ann Oncol 2003;14:123–30.

[17] de Wit M, Bohuslavizki KH, Buchert R, et al. 18FDG-PET following treatment as valid predictor for disease-free survival I Hodgkin's disease. Ann Oncol 2001;12:29–37.

[18] Naumann R, Vaic A, Beuthien-Baumann B, et al. Prognostic value of positron emission tomography in the evaluation of post-treatment residual mass in patients with Hodgkin's disease and non-Hodgkin's lymphoma. Br J Haematol 2001;115:793–800.

[19] Hueltenschmidt B, Sautter-Bihl ML, Lang O, et al. Whole body positron emission tomography in the treatment of Hodgkin disease. Cancer 2001;91:302–10.

[20] Guay C, Lepine M, Verreault J, et al. Prognostic value of PET using 18F-FDG in Hodgkin's disease for posttreatment evaluation. J Nucl Med 2003;44:1225–31.

[21] Spaepen K, Stroobants S, Dupont P, et al. Can positron emission tomography with [(18)F]-fluorodeoxyglucose after first-line treatment distinguish Hodgkin's disease patients who need additional therapy from others in whom additional therapy would mean avoidable toxicity? Br J Haematol 2001;115(2):272–8.

[22] Zijlstra JM, Lindauer-van der Werf G, Hoekstra OS, et al. 18F-fluoro-deoxyglucose positron emission tomography for post-treatment evaluation of malignant lymphoma: a systematic review. Haematologica 2006;91(4):522–9.

[23] Castellucci P, Nanni C, Farsad M, et al. Potential pitfalls of 18F-FDG PET in a large series of patients treated for malignant lymphoma: prevalence and scan interpretation. Nucl Med Commun 2005;26:689–94.

[24] Juweid ME, Stroobants S, Hoekstra OS, et al. Use of positron emission tomography (PET) for response assessment of lymphoma: consensus of the Imaging Subcommittee of International Harmonization Project (IHP) in lymphoma. J Clin Oncol 2007;25(5):571–8.

[25] Hutchings M, Mikhaeel NG, Fields PA, et al. Prognostic value of interim FDG-PET after two or three cycles of chemotherapy in Hodgkin lymphoma. Ann Oncol 2005;16(7):1160–8.

[26] Cheson BD, Pfistner B, Juweid ME, et al. Revised response criteria for malignant lymphoma. J Clin Oncol 2007;25(5):579–86.

[27] Reske SN. PET and restaging including residual masses and relapse. Eur J Nucl Med Mol Imaging 2003;30(Suppl 1):S89–96.

[28] Spaepen K, Stroobants S, Verhoef G, et al. Positron emission tomography with [(18)F]FDG for therapy response monitoring in lymphoma patients. Eur J Nucl Med Mol Imaging 2003;30(Suppl 1):S97–105.

[29] Freudenberg LS, Antoch G, Schütt P, et al. FDG-PET/CT in restaging of patients with lymphoma. Eur J Nucl Med Mol Imaging 2004;3:325–9.

[30] Schaefer NG, Hany TF, Taverna C, et al. Non-Hodgkin's lymphoma and Hodgkin's disease: coregistered FDG-PET and CT at staging and restaging—do we need contrast-enhanced CT? Radiology 2004;232:823–9.

[31] Raanani P, Shasha Y, Perry C, et al. Is CT still necessary for staging in Hodgkin and non-Hodgkin's lymphoma patients in the PET/CT era? Ann Oncol 2006;17:117–22.

[32] Palmedo H, Urbach H, Bender H, et al. FDG-PET in immunocompetent patients with primary central nervous system lymphoma: correlation with MRI and clinical follow-up. Eur J Nucl Med Mol Imaging 2006;33:164–8.

[33] Pakos EE, Fotopoulos AD, Ioannidis JP. 18F-FDG PET for evaluation of bone marrow infiltration in staging of lymphoma: a meta-analysis. J Nucl Med 2005;46(6):958–63.

[34] Diehl V, Franklin J, Pfreundschuh M, et al. Standard and increased-dose BEACOPP chemotherapy compared with COPP-ABVD for advanced Hodgkin's disease. N Engl J Med 2003;348(24):2386–95.

[35] Hasenclever D, Diehl V. International Prognostic Factors Project on Advanced Hodgkin's Disease. N Engl J Med 1998;339(21):1506–14.

[36] Gobbi PG, Zinzani PL, Broglia C, et al. Comparison of prognostic models in patients with advanced Hodgkin's disease. Cancer 2001;91:1467–78.

[37] Spaepen K, Stroobants S, Dupont P, et al. [(18)F]FDG PET monitoring of tumour response to chemotherapy: does [(18)F]FDG uptake correlate with the viable tumour cell fraction? Eur J Nucl Med Mol Imaging 2003;30(5):682–8.

[38] Römer W, Hanauske AR, Ziegler S, et al. Positron emission tomography in Non Hodgkin's lymphoma: assessment of chemotherapy with fluorodeoxyglucose. Blood 1998;91: 4464–71.

[39] Mikhaeel NG, Mainwaring P, Nunan T, et al. Prognostic value of interim and post treatment FDG-PET scanning in Hodgkin lymphoma [abstract]. Ann Oncol 2002;13(Suppl 2):21.

[40] Hutchings M, Loft A, Hansen M, et al. FDG-PET after two cycles of chemotherapy predicts treatment failure and progression-free survival in Hodgkin lymphoma. Blood 2006;107(1): 52–9.

[41] Gallamini A, Rigacci L, Merli F, et al. The predictive value of positron emission tomography scanning performed after two courses of standard therapy on treatment outcome in advanced stage Hodgkin's disease. Haematologica 2006;91(4):475–81.

[42] Kostakoglu L, Goldsmith SJ, Leonard JP, et al. FDG-PET after 1 cycle of therapy predicts outcome in diffuse large cell lymphoma and classic Hodgkin disease. Cancer 2006;107(11): 2678–87.

[43] Torizuka T, Nakamura F, Kanno T, et al. Early therapy monitoring with FDG-PET in aggressive non-Hodgkin's lymphoma and Hodgkin's lymphoma. Eur J Nucl Med Mol Imaging 2004;31(1):22–8.

[44] Dann EJ, Bar-Shalom R, Tamir A, et al. Risk-adapted BEACOPP regimen can reduce the cumulative dose of chemotherapy for standard and high-risk Hodgkin lymphoma with no impairment of outcome. Risk adapted BEACOPP regimen can reduce the cumulative dose of chemotherapy for standard and high risk Hodgkin lymphoma with no impairment of outcome. Blood 2007;109(3):905–9.

[45] Coleman M, Rafla S, Propert KJ, et al. Augmented therapy of extensive Hodgkin's disease: radiation to known disease or prolongation of induction chemotherapy did not improve survival–results of a cancer and leukemia Group B study. Int J Radiat Oncol Biol Phys 1998;41(3):639–45.

[46] Armitage JO, Weisenburger DD, Hutchins M, et al. Chemotherapy for diffuse large-cell lymphoma—rapidly responding patients have more durable remissions. J Clin Oncol 1986;4(2):160–4.

[47] Brice P, Bouabdallah R, Moreau P, et al. Prognostic factors for survival after high-dose therapy and autologous stem cell transplantation for patients with relapsing Hodgkin's disease: analysis of 280 patients from the French registry. Societe Francaise de Greffe de Moelle. Bone Marrow Transplant 1997;20(1):21–6.

[48] Becherer A, Mitterbauer M, Jaeger U, et al. Positron emission tomography with [18F]2-fluoro-D-2-deoxyglucose (FDG-PET) predicts relapse of malignant lymphoma after high-dose therapy with stem cell transplantation. Leukemia 2002;16(2):260–7.

[49] Cremerius U, Fabry U, Wildberger JE, et al. Pre-transplant positron emission tomography (PET) using fluorine-18-fluoro-deoxyglucose (FDG) predicts outcome in patients treated with high-dose chemotherapy and autologous stem cell transplantation for non-Hodgkin's lymphoma. Bone Marrow Transplant 2002;30:103–11.

[50] Filmont JE, Czernin J, Yap C, et al. Value of F-18 fluorodeoxyglucose positron emission tomography for predicting the clinical outcome of patients with aggressive lymphoma prior to and after autologous stem-cell transplantation. Chest 2003;124:608–13.

[51] Spaepen K, Stroobants S, Dupont P, et al. Prognostic value of pretransplantation positron emission tomography using fluorine 18-fluorodeoxyglucose in patients with aggressive

lymphoma treated with high-dose chemotherapy and stem cell transplantation. Blood 2003;102:53–9.

[52] Svoboda J, Andreadis C, Elstrom R, et al. Prognostic value of FDG-PET scan imaging in lymphoma patients undergoing autologous stem cell transplantation. Bone Marrow Transplant 2006;38(3):211–6.

[53] Schot BW, Zijlstra JM, Sluiter WJ, et al. Early FDG-PET assessment in combination with clinical risk scores determines prognosis in recurring lymphoma. Blood 2007;109(2):486–91.

[54] Schot BW, Pruim J, van Imhoff GW, et al. The role of serial pre-transplantation positron emission tomography in predicting progressive disease in relapsed lymphoma. Haematologica 2006;91(4):490–5.

New Strategies for the Treatment of Early Stages of Hodgkin's Lymphoma

David A. Macdonald, MD[a], Joseph M. Connors, MD[b,c,*]

[a]Division of Hematology, QEII Health Sciences Centre, Room 430, Bethune Building, 1278 Tower Road, Halifax, Nova Scotia B3H 2Y9, Canada
[b]University of British Columbia, Vancouver, British Columbia, Canada
[c]Lymphoma Tumour Group, British Columbia Cancer Agency, 600 West 10th Avenue, Vancouver, British Columbia V5Z 4E6, Canada

The last century has seen a remarkable evolution in the treatment of Hodgkin's lymphoma, in particular for patients diagnosed with limited-stage disease. The identification of the responsiveness of this disease to radiotherapy at the turn of the twentieth century led to early attempts to cure the disease with high doses delivered to known disease sites in a single fraction [1]; however, it was not until the 1950s that long-term survivals and possible cures were reported using daily, fractionated radiotherapy delivered not only to involved sites but also to adjacent nodal regions [2,3].

Although excellent results were being seen with wide-field radiotherapy techniques, three important observations began to emerge: (1) relapses after radiotherapy were occurring in about 25% of patients, almost always outside the radiation fields, indicating the presence of undetectable, micrometastatic disease at the time of original diagnosis [4]; (2) clinically significant long-term toxicities of radiotherapy emerged, including cardiovascular disease and second malignancies [5]; (3) even as curative strategies of radiotherapy were developed for limited-stage disease, chemotherapeutic agents effective in advanced-stage Hodgkin's lymphoma were developed. In 1967 DeVita and coworkers [6] reported that a combination of drugs with partially nonoverlapping toxicities, given in 28-day cycles (the MOPP regimen [mechlorethamine, vincristine, procarbazine and prednisone]), could cure about one half of patients who had advanced-stage disease. Over the next three decades, building on the observation of the curative potential of radiation and multiagent chemotherapy, combined modality therapy has emerged as the standard of care for limited-stage Hodgkin's lymphoma. Because systemic chemotherapy can reduce out-of-field relapses by treating micrometastatic disease, thereby also eliminating the requirement for staging laparotomy, it has made possible an era of clinical

*Corresponding author. Lymphoma Tumour Group, British Columbia Cancer Agency, 600 West 10th Avenue, Vancouver, British Columbia V5Z 4E6, Canada. E-mail address: jconnors@bccancer.bc.ca (J.M. Connors).

0889-8588/07/$ – see front matter
doi:10.1016/j.hoc.2007.06.014
© 2007 Elsevier Inc. All rights reserved.
hemonc.theclinics.com

investigation exploring the use of reduced radiation doses and fields in an effort to reduce the long-term toxicities without sacrificing overall disease control. Current and future investigations are now taking these observations a step further by evaluating strategies that treat most patients with limited-stage Hodgkin's lymphoma with multiagent chemotherapy alone, reserving radiotherapy only for those who would be destined to relapse without it.

DEFINITION OF LIMITED-STAGE HODGKIN'S LYMPHOMA

Hodgkin's lymphoma continues to be staged according to the Cotswolds modifications of the Ann Arbor staging system [7]. For the purpose of treatment algorithms, and in particular for defining patient populations for clinical trials, the classification is simplified to divide patients into limited stage, which was in the past treated with extended-field radiotherapy, or advanced stage, which required multiagent chemotherapy to provide a chance of cure. Staging laparotomy was previously used to better define the population that had disease truly limited to the supradiaphragmatic regions, but this has less usefulness when combined-modality therapy is used for limited-stage disease, presumably because of effective eradication of micrometastatic disease by the chemotherapy [8].

In North America, limited-stage disease is defined as stage I or IIA with no areas of bulk, defined as a mass greater than 10 cm. This definition represents approximately 30% to 40% of newly diagnosed patients [9]. Patients who have B symptoms or bulky disease are believed to have clinical course similar to those who have stage III–IV disease and are treated with full courses of chemotherapy, with radiation therapy considered for sites of initial bulk, particularly mediastinal. European cooperative groups have defined a group of patients who have intermediate risk, described as early-stage unfavorable. This group includes patients who are stage I–II with one or more of: age greater than 50, B symptoms, bulky mediastinal disease, elevated erythrocyte sedimentation rate, or four or more involved sites [10].

COMBINED MODALITY THERAPY AS STANDARD OF CARE

Peters and Kaplan [2,3] are credited with demonstrating much of the early success of wide-field radiation for limited-stage Hodgkin's lymphoma nearly five decades ago. Retrospective studies have addressed the question of adequate dose [11], but the only prospective trial of radiotherapy alone was a German Hodgkin's Lymphoma Study Group (GHSG) trial that compared 40 Gy of extended-field radiotherapy (EFRT) to 30 Gy of EFRT with additional 10 Gy to involved fields (IFRT) [12]. This multicenter randomized trial included 376 patients who had laparotomy-proven stage I–IIB disease without risk factors, and showed no difference between the arms, with 5-year freedom from treatment failure and overall survival of 76% and 97%, respectively. Attempts to reduce the radiation field to a supradiaphragmatic mantle field, even when limited to favorable patients with low risk for abdominal disease, have generally been disappointing [1].

The relapse rates observed using extended-field radiotherapy alone were 20% to 25% even after laparotomy-based staging. The next generation of clinical investigation combined radiotherapy with chemotherapy in an effort to improve disease control. Randomized trials established that relapse rates could be reduced to less than 10% by adding chemotherapy to EFRT, and this finding is supported by a large meta-analysis [4,13,14]. Toxicity remained an important drawback to combined modality treatment (CMT), leading to randomized trials attempting to reduce toxicity without sacrificing disease control or survival. Strategies included reduction of radiation fields, reduction of radiation doses, and reduction of number of cycles of chemotherapy. A detailed discussion of the details of all the clinical trials that addressed this question is beyond the scope of this article. The major trials are summarized in Table 1 [4,13,15–21]. In general, these trials demonstrated that disease control and survival were not compromised by these strategies. Longer-term follow-up is required to determine if late relapses will become an issue and to assess the effects on late toxicities, including second malignancies and cardiovascular disease.

Few direct comparisons of different chemotherapy regimens used as part of CMT for limited-stage Hodgkin's lymphoma have yet been published, none have used the doxorubicin, bleomycin, vinblastine, and dacarbazine (ABVD) regimen, which has been established as the standard of care in both advanced-stage and early-stage (unfavorable) disease [22,23]. Its favorable toxicity profile has resulted in its adoption as the standard chemotherapy used as part of CMT for limited-stage disease. The current GHSG HD13 trial is evaluating whether toxicity can be further reduced by the elimination of dacarbazine, bleomycin, or both when two cycles of chemotherapy are given followed by 30 Gy IFRT [24].

CHEMOTHERAPY ALONE FOR LIMITED-STAGE HODGKIN'S LYMPHOMA

Chemotherapy alone has been the subject of investigation for limited-stage Hodgkin's lymphoma in a small number of randomized trials. Several of these studies used chemotherapy regimens other than ABVD: the Grupo Argentino de Tratamiento de la Leucemia Aguda (GATLA) and Grupo Latinoamericano de Tratamiento de Hematopatías Malignas (GLATHEM) studied six cycles of CVPP followed by IFRT versus observation [25], and the European Organization for Research and Treatment of Cancer (EORTC) H9F three-armed trial randomized patients who achieved complete remission after six cycles of EBVP to 36 Gy IFRT, 20 Gy IFRT, or observation [21]. Although these studies produced encouraging results with chemotherapy alone they are of limited relevance today because they used chemotherapy regimens we now know are inferior to ABVD, leading to an underestimation of the disease control that can be achieved with uni-modality treatment.

A Spanish group prospectively treated 95 patients who had stage I or II Hodgkin's lymphoma with six cycles of ABVD without radiation and reported 7-year overall survival (OS) and progression-free survival (PFS) of 96% and 84%, respectively [26]. This study included patients who had B symptoms or bulky mediastinal disease, characteristics that other investigators have usually reserved to identify more advanced disease. This study was nonrandomized,

Table 1
Major trials examining questions relevant to the treatment of limited-stage Hodgkin's lymphoma

Trial	Treatment regimens	n	PFS	OS	Ref.
Clinical trials comparing EFRT to CT + EFRT					
GHSG HD7	EFRT 30 Gy (IFRT 40 Gy)	305	75	94	Sieber et al [4]
	2 ABVD + EFRT 30 Gy (IFRT 40 Gy)	312	91	94	
SWOG 9133/CALGB 9391	STLI (S) 36–40 Gy	163	81	96	Press et al [13]
	3 AV + STLI (S) 36–40 Gy	166	94	96	
Clinical trials comparing CT + IFRT to CT + EFRT					
Bonadonna	4 ABVD + STNI	66	93	96	Bondadonna et al [15]
	4 ABVD + IFRT	70	94	94	
Clinical trials comparing EFRT to CT + IFRT					
EORTC H7F	STNI	165	78	92	Noordijk et al [16]
	6 EBVP + STNI	168	88	92	
BNLI	Mantle RT 30–35 Gy (IFRT 30–40 Gy)	115	70	92	Radford et al [17]
	1 VAPEC-B + IFRT 30–40 Gy	111	87	98	
Stanford	STNI	43	92	n/a	Horning et al [18]
	VBM + IFRT	35	87	—	
EORTC/GELA H8F	STLI (S)	272	80	95	Hagenbeek et al [19]
	3 MOPP/ABV + IFRT 36 Gy	271	99	99	
Clinical trials of CMT comparing no. of cycles CT and/or dose of IFRT					
GHSG HD10	2 ABVD + IFRT 30 Gy	204	(A+B) 97	98	Diehl et al [20]
	2 ABVD + IFRT 20 Gy	210	(C+D) 96	99	
	4 ABVD + IFRT 30 Gy	218	(A+C) 97	99	
	4 ABVD + IFRT 20 Gy	215	(B+D) 98	99	
EORTC H9F	6 EBVP + IFRT 36 Gy	n/a	87	98	Noordijk et al [21]
	6 EBVP + IFRT 20 Gy	—	84	98	
	6 EBVP	—	70	98	

Abbreviations: ABVD, doxorubicin, bleomycin, vinblastine, and dacarbazine; BNLI, British National Lymphoma Investigation; CALGB, Cancer and Leukemia Group B; CMT, combined modality treatment; CT, chemotherapy; EBVP, epirubicin, bleomycin, vinblastine, and prednisone; EFRT, extended field radiotherapy; EORTC, European Organization for Research and Treatment of Cancer; GELA, Groupe d'Etude des Lymphomes de l'Adulte; GHSG, German Hodgkin's lymphoma Study Group; IFRT, involved field radiotherapy; MOPP, mechlorethamine, vincristine, procarbazine, and prednisone; n/a, not available; OS, overall survival; PFS, progression-free survival; STLI, subtotal lymphoid irradiation; STNI, subtotal nodal irradiation; SWOG, Southwest Oncology Group; VAPEC-B, doxorubicin, cyclophosphamide, vincristine, bleomycin, etoposide, prednisolone, and methotrexate; VBM, vinblastine, bleomycin, and methotrexate.

but the authors argue that the OS and PFS compare favourably to stage I–II patients receiving combined modality therapy on the EORTC H8 trials, in which 5-year OS and PFS were 94% and 86%, respectively [27].

Four randomized trials using ABVD or an equivalent chemotherapy regimen have evaluated chemotherapy alone versus chemotherapy followed by radiotherapy [22–25]. In a Children's Cancer Group trial (CCG 5942), 501 patients who achieved complete remission with risk-adapted chemotherapy were randomized to observation or IFRT [28]. The chemotherapy was four cycles of cyclophosphamide, vincristine, procarbazine, prednisone, doxorubicin, bleomycin, and vinblastine (COPP-ABV) for Stage I–IIA patients who did not have adverse risk factors, six cycles of COPP-ABV for stage I–III patients who had adverse risk factors or B symptoms, and an intensification of COPP-ABV with high-dose cytarabine and etoposide for stage IV patients. For all treated patients, 3-year event-free survival (EFS) favored those who received radiotherapy, but there was no difference in overall survival (3-year EFS 92% and 3-year OS 98% for chemotherapy plus radiation; 87% and 99% for chemotherapy alone, respectively). For the 42% of patients who had limited-stage lymphoma, 3-year EFS was 97% after IFRT and 91% without radiation (*P* for subgroup not reported), but 3-year OS was 100% for both groups.

A trial conducted in India considered a similar question in 179 adult patients who had various stages of Hodgkin's lymphoma who achieved complete remission after six cycles of ABVD, then were randomized to IFRT or no further treatment [29]. This trial also showed improved 8-year EFS with the use of radiotherapy (88% for ABVD plus IFRT; 76% for ABVD alone; $P = .01$) but interestingly also showed an overall survival advantage (8-year OS 100% for ABVD plus IFRT, 89% for ABVD alone, $P = .002$). Interpretation of these results is complicated by the inclusion in this trial of both adult and pediatric patients, patients of all stages, patients who had bulky disease, and patients who had B symptoms. Subset analysis of 99 patients who had stage I–II disease showed no difference in 8-year EFS or OS with the addition of IFRT (97% versus 94%, $P = .29$, and 100% versus 98%, $P = .26$, respectively).

A trial conducted at Memorial Sloan-Kettering limited enrolled 152 adult patients who had stage I–IIIA non-bulky disease who were randomized to six cycles of ABVD versus the same chemotherapy plus IFRT [30]. Unlike the other trials, this one showed no significant difference in freedom from progression (FFP), but a trend toward a survival benefit with combined modality therapy. The trial only had sufficient power to detect differences greater than 20%, and the inclusion of stage IB, IIB, and IIIA makes application of the results less relevant to patients who have limited-stage disease.

For the various reasons described, the above trials did not answer the specific question of whether chemotherapy alone with ABVD is sufficient therapy for adult patients who have limited-stage Hodgkin's lymphoma. In 1994 the National Cancer Institute of Canada–Clinical Trials Group (NCIC-CTG), with the participation of the Eastern Cooperative Oncology Group, initiated a multicenter randomized controlled trial comparing a risk-adapted approach, including extended-field radiation therapy with or without ABVD, to an experimental arm using ABVD chemotherapy alone, for previously untreated limited-stage Hodgkin's lymphoma. The primary outcome was 12-year overall survival based on the hypothesis that an approach that avoided radiation would provide adequate disease control and improve long-term overall survival by decreasing the number of deaths attributable to cardiovascular disease and secondary neoplasms in the arm without radiation. Over the life of this trial standard radiation for the management of limited-stage Hodgkin's lymphoma changed from extended-field to involved-field radiation eventually making the "standard arm" of the trial no longer relevant. Because of this the trial was closed in 2005 and an initial analysis has been reported [31]. At a median follow-up of 4.2 years, there was no difference in estimated 5-year overall survival or event-free survival but the estimated 5-year freedom from disease progression modestly favored the radiation arm (93% versus 87%, $P = .006$). Interestingly, second cancers and cardiovascular events were already observed, with a trend to increased events in patients randomized to receive radiation therapy. These results suggest that with further follow-up, the original hypothesis of NCIC-CTG HD6 may be confirmed showing that overall survival will be reduced in the radiation-included arm because of excessive mortality from second cancers and cardiovascular disease.

The change in standard practice that brought about the early closure of the NCIC-CTG HD6 trial illustrates an important consideration for clinical trials in such a highly curable condition. The number of patients required to show significant improvements in survival, which is already expected to be greater than 90%, and the length of follow-up required to assess for fatal late toxicity of the treatments, create the risk that the standard arm will become obsolete during the lifetime of the trial. Despite this, the NCIC-CTG HD6 trial maintains its relevance as having the largest published cohort of adult limited-stage patients randomized to receive ABVD alone.

RESPONSE-ADAPTED THERAPY OF LIMITED-STAGE HODGKIN'S LYMPHOMA

In the NCIC-CTG HD.6 trial, patients randomized to chemotherapy alone underwent response assessment with CT scan after two cycles of ABVD. Thirty-five per cent of patients achieved complete remission (CR) or complete remission-unconfirmed (CRu). Those in complete remission received two additional cycles and those who did not achieve CR received four additional cycles. A subgroup analysis showed a significant difference in FFP between these groups (5-year estimates 95% versus 81%, respectively; $P = .007$). For the 69 patients randomized to chemotherapy alone who achieved a CR or CRu, the progression-free survival was similar to that for all patients randomized to treatment that included radiotherapy. Early complete response to chemotherapy, as assessed after two cycles of ABVD, may therefore be an important predictor for progression-free survival. The response as assessed by CT scanning does not do this well, however. In the NCIC CTG HD.6

trial 80% of patients who had less than a CR or CRu after two cycles of ABVD remained free of progression even though managed without radiation. Clearly, a better assessment tool is needed to identify patients who have a sufficiently high risk for relapse to justify a change in treatment to radiation.

As seen in HD.6, two thirds of patients who have limited-stage Hodgkin's lymphoma treated with chemotherapy alone have small but detectable residual masses on CT after two cycles of ABVD. CT scanning cannot distinguish fibrosis from persistent viable tumor; therefore a CT-based response-adapted strategy would result in overuse of radiotherapy. Positron emission tomography using glucose tagged with radioactive fluorine (FDG-PET), when used for posttherapy evaluation, is superior to CT for making this distinction, with excellent negative predictive value [32,33]. Recently, a small study has suggested that FDG-PET may even have excellent negative predictive value after just one cycle of ABVD [34]. Seventeen of 23 patients had a negative FDG-PET after one cycle of chemotherapy. All 17 also had a negative FDG-PET at the completion of therapy and remain in continued remission at the end of follow-up (range 17–38 months). This study included patients who had advanced disease. Of the 6 patients who had positive PET after one cycle, 4 had entered the study with advanced-stage disease. Based on this small study it is reasonable to estimate that only 10% to 20% of patients who have limited-stage Hodgkin's lymphoma will have a positive FDG-PET early in treatment with ABVD, and therefore a PET-based response-adapted strategy might avoid radiotherapy in 80% of patients who have limited-stage HL without sacrificing disease control.

Such a strategy of PET-based, response-adapted therapy has not yet been proven in a clinical trial. The current EORTC–Groupe d'Etude des Lymphomes de l'Adulte (GELA) H10 trial is evaluating this question in a large randomized trial. The standard arm involves three cycles of ABVD (favorable cohort) or four cycles (unfavorable cohort) followed by involved nodal radiotherapy (INRT). The experimental arm involves two cycles of ABVD followed by FDG-PET. PET-negative patients receive additional ABVD chemotherapy alone: two more cycles for favorable and four more for unfavorable. PET-positive patients receive two cycles of escalated BEACOPP followed by INRT. This trial recently started and has a target accrual of 1600 patients.

SUMMARY

Limited-stage Hodgkin's lymphoma is a highly curable disease with expected long-term disease-free and overall survival rates close to 90% and 95%, respectively. This success has come at a cost of long-term treatment-related toxicity, such that the newly diagnosed patient who lives beyond 10 to 15 years is more likely to die from late complications of treatment than from the disease itself. Efforts to improve survival must therefore endeavor to reduce toxicity without sacrificing long-term disease-specific survival. Combining chemotherapy and radiation allows a reduction of radiation field size and number of cycles of chemotherapy facilitating achievement of the goal of reducing late toxicity.

Because a strategy of two cycles of ABVD followed by involved-field radiation reduces the risks of secondary cancers and infertility while maintaining excellent disease control this approach has been widely adopted. To further reduce the risks of radiotherapy, chemotherapy with ABVD alone has been investigated and is emerging as a reasonable option for patients, recognizing that there may be some reduction in local disease control but that relapses in these patients can often be treated effectively. The next step in this ongoing evolution will be the use of highly predictive tools for response assessment, such as FDG-PET, to better define which small fraction of patients are destined to relapse after chemotherapy alone and thus are good candidates for the preemptive use of radiotherapy.

References

[1] Diehl V, Mauch PM, Harris NL. Hodgkin's disease. In: DeVita VT, Hellman S, Rosenberg SA, editors. Cancer: principles and practice of oncology. 6th edition. Philadelphia: Lippincott Williams & Wilkins; 2001. p. 2339–87.

[2] Peters MA. A study of survivals in Hodgkin's disease treated radiologically. AJR Am J Roentgenol 1950;63:299–311.

[3] Kaplan H. The radical radiotherapy of regionally localized Hodgkin's disease. Radiology 1962;78:553–61.

[4] Sieber M, Franklin J, Tesch H. Two cycles of ABVD plus extended field radiotherapy is superior to radiotherapy alone in early stage Hodgkin's disease: results of the German Hodgkin's Lymphoma Study Group (GHSG) Trial HD7. Paper presented at the American Society of Hematology, Philadelphia, December 8–12, 2002.

[5] Hoppe RT. Hodgkin's disease: complications of therapy and excess mortality. Ann Oncol 1997;8(Suppl 1):115–8.

[6] DeVita VT, Serpick AA. Combination chemotherapy in the treatment of advanced Hodgkin's disease. Proc Am Assoc Cancer Res 1967;8:13.

[7] Lister TA, Crowther D, Sutcliffe SB, et al. Report of a committee convened to discuss the evaluation and staging of patients with Hodgkin's disease: Cotswolds meeting. [published erratum appears in J Clin Oncol 1990 Sep;8(9):1602]. J Clin Oncol 1989; 7(11):1630–6.

[8] Carde P, Hagenbeek A, Hayat M, et al. Clinical staging versus laparotomy and combined modality with MOPP versus ABVD in early-stage Hodgkin's disease: the H6 twin randomized trials from the European Organization for Research and Treatment of Cancer Lymphoma Cooperative Group. J Clin Oncol 1993;11(11):2258–72.

[9] Connors JM. State-of-the-art therapeutics: Hodgkin's lymphoma. J Clin Oncol 2005;23(26): 6400–8.

[10] Diehl V, Thomas RK, Re D. Part II: Hodgkin's lymphoma—diagnosis and treatment. Lancet Oncol 2004;5(1):19–26.

[11] Vijayakumar S, Myrianthopoulos L. An updated dose-response analysis in Hodgkin's disease. Radiother Oncol 1992;24(1):1–13.

[12] Duhmke E, Diehl V, Loeffler M, et al. Randomized trial with early-stage Hodgkin's disease testing 30 Gy vs. 40 Gy extended field radiotherapy alone. Int J Radiat Oncol Biol Phys 1996;36(2):305–10.

[13] Press OW, LeBlanc M, Lichter AS, et al. Phase III randomized intergroup trial of subtotal lymphoid irradiation versus doxorubicin, vinblastine, and subtotal lymphoid irradiation for stage IA to IIA Hodgkin's disease. J Clin Oncol 2001;19(22):4238–44.

[14] Specht L, Gray RG, Clarke MJ, et al. Influence of more extensive radiotherapy and adjuvant chemotherapy on long-term outcome of early-stage Hodgkin's disease: a meta-analysis of

23 randomized trials involving 3,888 patients. International Hodgkin's Disease Collaborative Group. J Clin Oncol 1998;16(3):830–43.

[15] Bonadonna G, Bonfante V, Viviani S, et al. ABVD plus subtotal nodal versus involved-field radiotherapy in early-stage Hodgkin's disease: long-term results. J Clin Oncol 2004; 22(14):2835–41.

[16] Noordijk EM, Carde P, Dupouy N, et al. Combined-modality therapy for clinical stage I or II Hodgkin's lymphoma: long-term results of the European Organisation for Research and Treatment of Cancer H7 Randomized Controlled Trials. J Clin Oncol 2006;24(19): 3128–35.

[17] Radford J, Williams M, Hancock B. Minimal initial chemotherapy plus involved field radiotherapy (RT) versus mantle field RT for clinical stage I/IIA supradiaphragmatic Hodgkin's disease (HD). Results of the UK Lymphoma Group LY07 trial. Br J Cancer 2004;91(Suppl 1): S1–2 [abstract CT1].

[18] Horning SJ, Hoppe RT, Mason J, et al. Stanford-Kaiser Permanente G1 study for clinical stage I to IIA Hodgkin's disease: subtotal lymphoid irradiation versus vinblastine, methotrexate, and bleomycin chemotherapy and regional irradiation. J Clin Oncol 1997;15(5): 1736–44.

[19] Hagenbeek A, Eghbali H, Fermé C, et al. Three cycles of MOPP/ABV hybrid and involved-field irradiation is more effective than subtotal nodal irradiation in favorable supradiaphragmatic clinical stages I–II Hodgkin's disease: preliminary results of the EORTC-GELA H8-F randomized trial in 543 patients. Blood 2000;96:575a.

[20] Diehl V, Brillant C, Engert A, et al. HD10: investigating reduction of combined modality treatment intensity in early stage Hodgkin's lymphoma. Interim analysis of a randomized trial of the German Hodgkin Study Group (GHSG). J Clin Oncol (Meeting Abstracts) 2005;23(Suppl 16):6506.

[21] Noordijk EM, Thomas J, Ferme C, et al. First results of the EORTC-GELA H9 randomized trials: the H9-F trial (comparing 3 radiation dose levels) and H9-U trial (comparing 3 chemotherapy schemes) in patients with favorable or unfavorable early stage Hodgkin's lymphoma (HL). J Clin Oncol (Meeting Abstracts) 2005;23(Suppl 16): 6505.

[22] Canellos GP, Anderson JR, Propert KJ, et al. Chemotherapy of advanced Hodgkin's disease with MOPP, ABVD, or MOPP alternating with ABVD. N Engl J Med 1992;327(21): 1478–84.

[23] Diehl V, Brillant C, Engert A, et al. Recent interim analysis of the HD11 trial of the GHSG: intensification of chemotherapy and reduction of radiation dose in early unfavorable stage Hodgkin's lymphoma. Blood 2005;106(11):[abstract #816].

[24] Diehl V, Stein H, Hummel M, et al. Hodgkin's lymphoma: biology and treatment strategies for primary, refractory, and relapsed disease. Hematology: Am Soc Hematol Educ Program Book 2003;225–47.

[25] Duhmke E, Connors JM, Pavlovsky S, et al. Treatment of clinical stage I-II Hodgkin's disease. In: Mauch PM, Armitage JO, Diehl V, et al, editors. Hodgkin's disease. Philadelphia: Lippincott Williams & Wilkins; 1999. p. 435.

[26] Rueda Dominguez A, Marquez A, Guma J, et al. Treatment of stage I and II Hodgkin's lymphoma with ABVD chemotherapy: results after 7 years of a prospective study. Ann Oncol 2004;15(12):1798–804.

[27] Henry-Amar M, Meerwaldt JH, Carde P. The EORTC treatment strategy in Hodgkin's lymphoma: a 4-decade experience. Leuk Lymphoma 2001;42(Suppl 2):54.

[28] Nachman JB, Sposto R, Herzog P, et al. Randomized comparison of low-dose involved-field radiotherapy and no radiotherapy for children with Hodgkin's disease who achieve a complete response to chemotherapy. J Clin Oncol 2002;20(18):3765–71.

[29] Laskar S, Gupta T, Vimal S, et al. Consolidation radiation after complete remission in Hodgkin's disease following six cycles of doxorubicin, bleomycin, vinblastine, and dacarbazine chemotherapy: is there a need? J Clin Oncol 2004;22(1):62–8.

[30] Straus DJ, Portlock CS, Qin J, et al. Results of a prospective randomized clinical trial of doxo-rubicin, bleomycin, vinblastine, and dacarbazine (ABVD) followed by radiation therapy (RT) versus ABVD alone for stages I, II, and IIIA nonbulky Hodgkin disease. Blood 2004;104(12):3483–9.

[31] Meyer RM, Gospodarowicz MK, Connors JM, et al. Randomized comparison of ABVD che-motherapy with a strategy that includes radiation therapy in patients with limited-stage Hodgkin's lymphoma: National Cancer Institute of Canada Clinical Trials Group and the Eastern Cooperative Oncology Group. J Clin Oncol 2005;23(21):4634–42.

[32] de Wit M, Bohuslavizki KH, Buchert R, et al. 18FDG-PET following treatment as valid predic-tor for disease-free survival in Hodgkin's lymphoma. Ann Oncol 2001;12(1):29–37.

[33] Rigacci L, Castagnoli A, Dini C, et al. 18FDG-positron emission tomography in post treat-ment evaluation of residual mass in Hodgkin's lymphoma: long-term results. Oncol Rep 2005;14(5):1209–14.

[34] Kostakoglu L, Goldsmith SJ, Leonard JP, et al. FDG-PET after 1 cycle of therapy predicts out-come in diffuse large cell lymphoma and classic Hodgkin disease. Cancer 2006;107(11): 2678–87.

Do We Need an Early Unfavorable (Intermediate) Stage of Hodgkin's Lymphoma?

Lena Specht, MD, Phd[a],*, John Raemaekers, MD, Phd[b]

[a]Departments of Oncology and Haematology, The Finsen Centre, Rigshospitalet,
Copenhagen University Hospital, 9 Blegdamsvej, 2100 Copenhagen, Denmark
[b]Department of Medicine, Division of Hematology, University Hospital of Nijmegen,
P.O. Box 9101, Nijmegen HB 6500, The Netherlands

The Ann Arbor staging system for lymphomas remains the universally accepted system for categorizing patients who have Hodgkin's lymphoma [1]. Patients who have stage I/II disease are generally considered early stage, whereas patients who have stage III/IV are considered to have advanced-stage disease. There is not complete consensus on this issue, however, as some consider stage IIB advanced and some consider stage IIIA early.

Prediction of outcome by prognostic factors is important because patients may be separated accordingly into risk groups determining treatment selection. The Ann Arbor staging system cannot be relied on as the only prognostic tool in Hodgkin's lymphoma, however. Many other features of prognostic importance have become recognized, many of them related to the extent and volume of disease. The extent of disease may vary considerably in stages other than stage I, and the volume of disease in individual regions is not taken into account at all in the Ann Arbor classification. The Cotswold modification of the staging system incorporates a designation for number of sites and bulk [2], but this modification has not been universally adopted. Numerous other prognostic factors for different Ann Arbor stages, presentations, treatments, and outcomes have been examined, and varying combinations of some of these factors are presently being used by different centers and groups worldwide [3,4].

DEFINITION OF INTERMEDIATE (EARLY UNFAVORABLE) STAGE

In early-stage disease a separation into favorable and unfavorable (intermediate-stage) disease based on the absence or presence of certain risk factors has been used by various groups for patient stratification in clinical trials. The classification systems used by the German Hodgkin's Study Group (GHSG), the

*Corresponding author. E-mail address: lena.specht@rh.regionh.dk (L. Specht).

0889-8588/07/$ – see front matter
doi:10.1016/j.hoc.2007.07.002

© 2007 Elsevier Inc. All rights reserved.
hemonc.theclinics.com

European Organization for Research and Treatment of Cancer (EORTC), and the National Cancer Institute of Canada (NCIC) are shown in Table 1. The risk factors and prognostic groups were originally defined in the context of treatment with radiotherapy alone. In a combined-modality setting the difference in prognosis between favorable and unfavorable disease is expected to be smaller. Moreover, in more recent series treatment had been tailored according to the prognostic groups, and it is therefore not surprising that the risk factors had little independent significance [5].

RISK GROUPS IN THE CONTEXT OF PRESENT-DAY TREATMENT

The treatment of Hodgkin's lymphoma has improved dramatically over the past decades. The large majority of patients who have early-stage disease are cured by standard first-line combined-modality treatment. New dose-intensified chemotherapy regimens are even more efficient [6,7]. With increasing efficacy of primary treatment the importance of prognostic factors with regard to tumor control may diminish or even vanish, if practically all patients are cured. Intensification of treatment comes at a price, however. Long-term toxicity is now a major concern for patients who have early-stage Hodgkin's lymphoma. The long-term consequences of extensive radiotherapy, particularly with regard to second malignancies and cardiovascular disease, have been known

Table 1
Definition of favorable and unfavorable (intermediate) early-stage Hodgkin's lymphoma

	GHSG	EORTC	NCIC
Risk factors	Large mediastinal mass Extranodal disease ESR $\geq$50 without B symptoms or $\geq$30 with B symptoms $\geq$3 nodal areas	Large mediastinal mass Age $\geq$50 years ESR $\geq$50 without B symptoms or $\geq$30 with B symptoms $\geq$4 nodal areas	Histology other than LP/NS Age $\geq$40 years ESR $\geq$50 $\geq$3 nodal areas
Favorable	CS I/II without risk factors	CS I/II (supradiaphragmatic) without risk factors	CS I/II without risk factors
Unfavorable	CS I or CS IIA with $\geq$1 risk factor CS IIB with ESR $\geq$50 without B symptoms or $\geq$30 with B symptoms or $\geq$3 nodal areas but without large mediastinal mass and extranodal disease	CS I/II (supradiaphragmatic) with $\geq$1 risk factors	CS I/II with $\geq$1 risk factors

Abbreviations: CS, clinical stage; EORTC, European Organization for Research and Treatment of Cancer; ESR, erythrocyte sedimentation rate; GHSG, German Hodgkin's Lymphoma Study Group; LP, lymphocyte predominance; NCIC, National Cancer Institute of Canada; NS, nodular sclerosis.

for some time [8–21]. With long-term follow-up data on patients treated with modern chemotherapy regimens now becoming available it is evident that this modality also carries significant risks of late mortality and morbidity [6,13,19,21–28].

The goal of the treatment of early-stage Hodgkin's lymphoma is therefore no longer merely to cure the patients. The goal is now to cure the patients with as little treatment as possible to minimize the risk for treatment-related morbidity and mortality, but without jeopardizing the chance of cure of the Hodgkin's lymphoma. At first glance, one possible solution to this problem could be to give minimal treatment up front and then give salvage treatment to those who relapse. Long-term follow-up of randomized trials clearly show that this is not a viable solution, however. Patients who relapse receive intensive treatment, and the long-term consequence is a significantly increased risk for second malignancies and possibly other complications, which overshadows the possible benefits for the patients who do not relapse [10,11,29–31]. It is therefore mandatory to give adequate treatment up front to minimize the risk for relapse. To achieve this goal we need to be able to tailor the treatment to the individual patient, adjusting the intensity of treatment to that patient's risk profile. The division of early-stage patients into favorable and unfavorable (ie, intermediate stage) is, therefore, as relevant as ever. The purpose of dividing the patients in risk groups is not to find patients who have different outcomes, but to be able to tailor treatment to patients to achieve the same high cure rate for all patients with minimal toxicity.

UNFAVORABLE (INTERMEDIATE) STAGE VERSUS FAVORABLE EARLY-STAGE DISEASE

The clinical significance of separating the early favorable and unfavorable stages I and II is clearly demonstrated in the results of the EORTC H7 trial [32]. In this randomized controlled clinical trial the classic EORTC prognostic factors were used to identify patients for the favorable and the unfavorable arms. The strength of the study design is found in the experimental treatment arm being similar in both prognostic subsets of patients. This similarity allowed for a comparison with the standard treatment in each subset, independent of the prognostic factor score. The study was performed in the period between 1988 and 1993. As their standard treatment patients who had favorable characteristics received subtotal nodal irradiation (STNI); those in the unfavorable subset received six monthly cycles of the hybrid combination of MOPP/ABV (mechlorethamine, vincristine, procarbazine, prednisone, adriamycin, bleomycin, vinblastine and dacarbazine) followed by involved-field radiotherapy (IF-RT). The experimental arm consisted of a more easily tolerated and presumably less toxic variant of the ABVD regimen, namely EBVP (epirubicin, bleomycin, vinblastine, and prednisone). This schedule, first reported by Hoerni and colleagues [33], was given once every 3 weeks for a total of six cycles. The chemotherapy was followed by IF-RT at a dose of 36 to 40 Gy. In the favorable subset, 333 patients were enrolled. After a median follow-up of 9 years the EBVP regimen proved to be superior to the STNI in event-free survival (EFS): 88% versus 78% (10-year EFS, $P = .0113$). In the unfavorable group of 389 patients, however, the EBVP regimen was significantly inferior to the MOPP/ABV arm: 10-year EFS of 68% versus 88% ($P < .001$) and 10-year overall survival (OS) of 79% and 87% ($P = .0175$), respectively. A closer look at the data reveals that in the unfavorable subset during EBVP more progressions and after EBVP more relapses occurred as compared with MOPP/ABV. Relapses after EBVP occurred more often in initially irradiated and in nonirradiated areas. This finding suggests that, whereas in favorable patients EBVP was not associated with an increased number of progressions or relapses, EBVP is not strong enough in patients who have unfavorable prognostic characteristics.

This study is the only large randomized trial that really addressed the question of whether the classic prognostic factors, defined in the era of staging laparotomy and wide-field RT, are still valid for the modern combined-modality treatment approaches. Based on these results, it is justified to conclude that patients who have favorable and unfavorable early stages of disease should be treated as separate entities, because they need a different treatment intensity to reach high survival rates. The results of the GHSG HD10 and HD11 trials can be interpreted in the same way [34]. Although there was no identical experimental treatment arm in these trials for patients who had early favorable stages (HD10) and for those who had intermediate stages (HD11), as was the case in the EORTC H7 trial, and thus the two trials were not designed to test the significance of the prognostic factors, the treatment consisting of four cycles of ABVD followed by IF-RT was applied in both studies. In the favorable subset of patients, two cycles of ABVD proved to be as good as four cycles of ABVD, whereas in the unfavorable subset four cycles of ABVD was as effective as four cycles of BEACOPP baseline, showing that intensification of ABVD by BEACOPP baseline did not improve results.

UNFAVORABLE EARLY (INTERMEDIATE) STAGE IN RECENT PROTOCOLS AND TRIALS

The introduction of combined-modality approaches has resulted in a consistent improvement of prognosis. Progression-free survival (PFS) and OS of the patients who have unfavorable characteristics now approach that of the favorable subset. The more recent randomized clinical trials on early unfavorable stages mostly addressed further refinement of the treatment, be it defining the optimal chemotherapy schedule, the optimal number of chemotherapy cycles, or the extent and dose of RT. A summary of the trials is given in Table 2 [32,35–41]. PFS and OS rates consistently reach 85% to greater than 90%. The results underline the success of the modern combined-modality approach. ABVD is the accepted standard chemotherapy [42–44]. A minimum of four cycles of ABVD followed by IF-RT at a dose of 30 Gy with a boost of 6 Gy in case of PR after chemotherapy can be considered standard treatment at present. Probably, the dose of RT can be reduced to 20 Gy if the interim results of the GHSG HD11 trial still hold after more prolonged observation periods [36]. The EORTC H7 study has clearly demonstrated that a less intense chemotherapy schedule like EBVP unacceptably lowers remission and PFS rates [32]. It is unlikely, therefore, that reducing chemotherapy burden, aiming at reduction of toxicity, will result in maintaining the outcome at the high level of current standard treatment. This finding is corroborated by the results of the GOELAMS (Groupe Ouest-Est d'Étude des Leucémies et Autres Maladies du Sang) H90-NM study [45]. In this randomized trial, 386 patients were enrolled. Both early favorable and unfavorable patients were included. ABVDm (methylprednisolone) was compared with the potentially less toxic epirubicin, bleomycin, vinblastine, methotrexate, methylprednisolone (EBVMm), followed by extended-field radiotherapy (EF-RT) in responding patients. The ABVDm arm proved superior to the EBVMm treatment in complete remission rates and freedom from progression (FFP).

Some 10% to 15% of patients still fail the current standard. One could easily argue for a more intensive approach. This question was addressed in the EORTC/GELA (Groupe d'Etudes des Lymphomes de l'Adulte) H8U and H9U trials comparing different numbers of cycles of chemotherapy and a comparison between ABVD and BEACOPP baseline. Apparently, increasing the number of cycles from four to six or substituting BEACOPP baseline for ABVD does not improve the outcome. Comparable results have been reported from the GHSG HD5 and HD11 studies. Although escalated BEACOPP has proven its superiority in advanced stages of disease [6], there are no firm data yet to support its use in unfavorable early stages. Possibly, the recently started EORTC/GELA/IIL Intergroup H10 study will shed some light on the merits of escalated BEACOPP in patients who have early stages of disease who do not respond favorably to the first two cycles of ABVD (see later discussion). The other ongoing randomized trial addressing increasing intensity of chemotherapy is the NCI/SWOG (National Cancer Institute/South West Oncology Group) study comparing ABVD with the Stanford V schedule, though the selection of eligible patients is not identical to the definition of unfavorable early stages. Several other randomized studies have been completed with inclusion of, among other subsets, unfavorable intermediate stages [46–48]. These studies were designed to compare combined-modality treatment with chemotherapy only. Because of the mixture of different prognostic subsets of patients it is impossible to draw conclusions from these trials for the optimal treatment of the unfavorable early-stage patients.

INTERMEDIATE-STAGE VERSUS ADVANCED DISEASE WITH FAVORABLE PROGNOSTIC FACTORS

The question then arises as to why the early unfavorable or intermediate stages I and II patients should not be included in the groups of advanced-stage patients. Using the International Prognostic Score (IPS) for advanced-stage patients [49], patients who have stage III or IV disease can be divided into a good-risk group (zero, one, or two adverse prognostic factors) and a poor-risk group (three or more adverse factors). For the good-risk patients ABVD

Table 2
Recent randomized clinical trials in unfavorable stages I/II Hodgkin's lymphoma

Trial (reference)	Treatment	No. of patients	PFS (y)	OS (y)	Remarks
Extent and dose of RT					
GHSG HD8 [37]	A. COPP/ABVD × 2 + EF-RT 30–40 Gy	532	85% (5)	90% (5)	n.s.
	B. COPP/ABVD × 2 + IF-RT 30–40 Gy	532	84% (5)	92% (5)	
EORTC/GELA H8U [38]	A. MOPP/ABV × 6 + IF-RT 36–40 Gy	336	84% (7)	89% (7)	EFS instead of PFS; n.s.
	B. MOPP/ABV × 4 + IF-RT 36–40 Gy	333	86% (7)	90% (7)	
	C. MOPP/ABV × 4 + STNI 36–40 Gy	327	86% (7)	90% (7)	
Anselmo et al [35]	A. ABVD × 4 + EF-RT	102	94% (5)	97% (5)	n.s.
	B. ABVD × 4 + IFRT	107	91% (5)	96% (5)	
GHSG HD11 [36]	A. ABVD × 4 + IF-RT 30 Gy	327	87% (3)	96% (3)	Not final analysis; n.s.
	B. ABVD × 4 + IF-RT 20 Gy	325			
	C. BEACOPP × 4 + IF-RT 30 Gy	319			
	D. BEACOPP × 4 + IF-RT 20 Gy	329			
Chemotherapy: number of cycles					
EORTC/GELA H8U [38]	See above	—	—	—	—

Study	Treatment	n	EFS/FFTF (y)	OS (y)	Comments
EORTC/GELA H9U [39]	A. ABVD × 6 + IF-RT 30–36 Gy	276	91% (4)	95% (4)	Not final analysis; EFS instead of PFS; n.s.
	B. ABVD × 4 + IF-RT 30–36 Gy	277	87% (4)	94% (4)	
	C. BEACOPP × 4 + IF-RT 30–36 Gy	255	90% (4)	93% (4)	
Chemotherapy: schedule					
GHSG HD5 [41]	A. COPP/ABVD × 2 + EF-RT 30–40 Gy	487	80% (7)	88% (7)	n.s.
	B. COPP/ABV/IMEP × 2 + EF-RT 30–40 Gy	486	79% (7)	88% (7)	
EORTC H7U [32]	A. MOPP/ABV × 6 + IF-RT 36–40 Gy	195	88% (10)	87% (10)	EFS instead of PFS; EFS P<.001; OS P=.0175
	B. EBVP × 6 + IF-RT 36–40 Gy	194	68% (10)	79 (10)	
GHSG HD11 [36]	See above	—	—	—	—
EORTC/GELA H9U [39]	See above	—	—	—	—
Chemotherapy: no RT					
NCIC/ECOG [40] excluding bulky disease	A. ABVD × 2 + STNI 35 Gy	139	95% (5)	92% (5)	PFS P=.004; OS n.s.
	B. ABVD × 4–6 no RT	137	88% (5)	95% (5)	

Abbreviations: ECOG, Eastern Cooperative Oncology Group; EF-RT, extended-field radiotherapy; EFS, event-free survival; EORTC, European Organization for Research and Treatment of Cancer; GELA, Groupe d'Etudes des lymphomes de l'Adulte; GHSG, German Hodgkin's Study Group; IF-RT, involved-field radiotherapy; NCIC, National Cancer Institute of Canada; n.s., statistically not significant; OS, overall survival; PFS, progression-free survival; RT, radiotherapy; STNI, subtotal nodal irradiation.

is standard chemotherapy for a total of six to eight cycles. Those who reach a CR after four cycles of ABVD can be treated effectively with six cycles, whereas those who reach the CR only after six cycles need a total of eight cycles [50]. There is compelling evidence that for the patients who have good-risk stage III/IV disease who reach a CR on chemotherapy, additional IF-RT is not indicated, although not all agree [51–62]. Advanced-stage patients who do not reach CR but only a PR on six cycles of adequate chemotherapy have excellent survival rates when additional IF-RT is given [63]. Following this strategy for advanced-stage patients, the FFS and OS rates of 80% to 90%, respectively, are similar to those of the patients who have unfavorable early stages. This finding offers a good rationale to include the patients who have unfavorable early stages in new trials for patients who have good-risk advanced stages of disease.

It is not that obvious, however. For patients who have unfavorable early stages, combined-modality treatment is still the undisputed standard treatment, whereas for those who have good-risk advanced disease chemotherapy alone is sufficient treatment for 60% to 70% of the patients. Combining both subsets of patients into one group would imply that the good-risk advanced-stage patients would again be treated with a combined-modality approach. Because these patients by definition have disease activity on both sides of the diaphragm, radiation fields can become extensive. That is clearly in contradiction with our aims to reduce long-term toxicity and it neglects the good results of chemotherapy alone.

FUTURE ASPECTS

Are there any new prognostic markers that can be of help to identify subsets of patients within the unfavorable early stages who need more aggressive treatment and those who could be treated less intensively? The EORTC prognostic criteria or the slightly modified EORTC criteria as used by the GHSG still are the easiest to use and most clinically relevant markers.

The IPS developed for patients who have advanced-stage disease has been tested for its applicability in 1424 patients who had early-stage disease enrolled in the GHSG HD4 and HD5 trials [64]. Only the factor low albumin gave a significant contribution to the usual clinical prognostic variables. A poor-risk subgroup of 20% of the patients had an 8% lower PFS at 6 years. In a series of 1156 patients enrolled by the GELA in the EORTC/GELA H8 and H9 study a comparable analysis has been performed [5]. There seemed to be some prognostic role for a combination of male gender, age >45 years, low hemoglobin and lymphocyte count, B symptoms with elevated ESR, and extranodal sites. As compared with the more classic criteria this new index did not add substantially in identifying specific risk groups. In conclusion, the modest additional predictive ability of the IPS does not justify its use in early-stage disease.

In a joint attempt of GHSG, EORTC, and GELA, six randomized trials concerning patients who had early-stage disease and risk factors were selected to identify factors that may predict a particularly poor prognosis within this subset [65]. Patients received four to six cycles of ABVD or ABVD-like chemotherapy plus radiotherapy. A total of 4490 patients were enrolled in the six selected trials. Male gender, older age, B symptoms, and mediastinal bulk were associated with greater risk for failure. Based on these factors it was estimated that about 20% of patients would experience a relatively poor PFS (eg, 76% 5-year PFS) compared with 84% to 92% in the remainder when treated with standard treatment. The important prognostic role of age in tolerability of treatment was once more highlighted by Klimm and colleagues [66]. Some other series failed also in improving the current EORTC/GHSG criteria [67,68]. These data suggest that improvement of treatment could be beneficial for a subgroup of patients who have early unfavorable disease, but we cannot identify this subset using the well-known clinical prognostic parameters.

New prognostic scores based on pretreatment clinical characteristics are unlikely to facilitate individually tailored treatment designs. The most promising new development is the use of positron emission tomography with fluorodeoxyglucose (FDG-PET scan) as an early indicator of treatment response. There is accumulating evidence that the result of a FDG-PET scan after two cycles of chemotherapy is highly predictive of the outcome of the prescheduled treatment. In the study by Hutchings and colleagues [69], the 61 patients who had a negative FDG-PET scan after two cycles of ABVD had a highly significantly better 2-year PFS than the 16 patients who had a positive scan: 96% versus 0% ($P < .001$). In the former only 3 of the 61 patients progressed during the median follow-up of 23 months; in the latter 11 of the 16 patients progressed. These are impressive results, but we should be careful in interpreting the results into clinical practice. First, it is not clear from the data to what degree these results are to be used in patients who have unfavorable stage I/II disease. The prognostic criteria were not identical to the EORTC or GHSG criteria. In the subgroup of 31 patients who had early-stage disease, 5 patients had a positive FDG-PET scan after two cycles of ABVD. Only one of these 5 patients progressed during follow-up. In the group of 26 patients who had a negative FDG-PET scan, none progressed. The negative predictive value thus seems to be much stronger in early-stage patients than the predictive value of a positive early FDG-PET scan. In addition, we have to bear in mind that a negative FDG-PET scan after two cycles of ABVD is not identical to cure. These patients all have received additional RT after the scheduled two to four cycles of ABVD. The finding of only one relapse in the 5 early FDG-PET scan–positive patients suggests that the completion of therapy with subsequent cycles of ABVD followed by RT was effective.

Similar results have been reported by Gallamini and colleagues [70]. In their multicenter study, 108 patients who had newly diagnosed Hodgkin's lymphoma were enrolled in a prospective evaluation of the predictive value of FDG-PET scanning after two courses of chemotherapy. The vast majority of patients received ABVD chemotherapy. Fifty-five percent of patients had stage IIA unfavorable or stage IIB disease; the remaining patients all had advanced stages of disease. In the whole group of 108 patients, 20 had a positive FDG-PET scan after two courses of chemotherapy, 17 of whom developed relapse or progressive disease. In contrast, 85 of the 88 patients who had a negative

FDG-PET scan after two courses remained in CR after a mean follow-up of 1 year. Unfortunately no data are given for specific subgroups separately (eg, the unfavorable early stages). Although follow-up is short, an early FDG-PET scan holds the promise to become a predictive marker of utmost clinical significance and usefulness in the design of individually tailored treatment approaches [71,72].

The new response criteria in Hodgkin's lymphoma incorporate the FDG-PET scan at the end of treatment in assessing remission status [73]. A pretreatment FDG-PET scan is strongly recommended. An interim FDG-PET scan (eg, after two cycles of chemotherapy) is considered to be experimental and only to be advised in the context of a clinical trial. It is encouraging that several cooperative groups have now launched randomized clinical trials in patients who have unfavorable early-stage disease incorporating an experimental arm that is FDG-PET scan result-driven.

The ongoing Intergroup H10 study of EORTC, GELA, and IIL (Intergruppo Italiano di Linfomi) for patients who have untreated stage I and II disease tests the adaptation of treatment according to the result of the early FDG-PET scan as opposed to giving the standard treatment without taking into account the result of the FDG-PET scan after two cycles of ABVD (study design, Fig. 1). In this trial the same policy of adapting treatment is followed in the favorable and the unfavorable groups of patients. As mentioned earlier for the EORTC H7 trial, this design offers the opportunity to test a new treatment

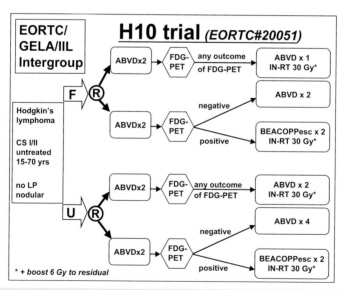

Fig. 1. Study design of the randomized controlled clinical EORTC/GELA/IIL Intergroup H10 trial on patients who have CS I/II Hodgkin's lymphoma. EORTC, European Organization for Research and Treatment of Cancer; GELA, Groupe d'Etudes des Lymphomes de l'Adulte; IIL, Intergruppo Italiano di Linfomi.

approach independent of the clinical pretreatment prognostic stratification. The main objective of the H10 trial is to reduce long-term toxicity of treatment by omitting RT in patients who have a negative FDG-PET scan after two cycles, the presumably good outcome group. Conversely, one might expect a 10% to 15% positive early FDG-PET scan rate in these cohorts of patients based on available literature data. When these 10% to 15% of patients are the ones that fail our current standard treatment, an early change of chemotherapy could possibly improve their outcome. We therefore intensify the treatment for this subset of patients in the experimental arm by switching from ABVD to escalated BEACOPP, still followed by RT, aiming at improvement of efficacy.

The NCRI Lymphoma Clinical Studies Group from the United Kingdom has embarked on a study for patients who have low-risk early-stage disease: after 3 cycles of ABVD, patients who have a negative FDG-PET scan are randomized between IF-RT and no further treatment; those who have a positive FDG-PET scan receive a fourth cycle of ABVD followed by IF-RT. The GHSG are preparing their new generation clinical trials in which early FDG-PET scans will take a prominent place for refining treatment approaches.

Another important new development is the modification of RT. A lower rate of late complications is expected with lower radiation doses. Smaller radiation fields should lead to a decrease in late effects. The increased efficacy of chemotherapy and the increased use of effective chemotherapy in patients who have early-stage disease calls for a reconsideration of the RT fields, because most of the presumed occult disease is eradicated by chemotherapy already. Modern imaging techniques, including better CT scan imaging and especially combined FDG-PET/CT scans, allow for a more precise delineation of the target tissue. Girinsky and colleagues [74] recently extensively illustrated the concept of involved-node RT (IN-RT) instead of IF-RT. The new IN-RT concept, which encompasses only the initially involved lymph nodes instead of the whole lymph node region, is now being applied in the EORTC/GELA/IIL Intergroup H10 study with the hope of achieving a high local control rate without long-term toxicity.

New biologic prognostic markers would be most welcome in identifying specific subsets of patients. A discussion of these markers is beyond the scope of this article, however.

SUMMARY

The outcome of patients who have early unfavorable or intermediate-stage Hodgkin's lymphoma has greatly improved. The standard treatment is combined-modality treatment consisting of a fixed number of chemotherapy cycles (generally four cycles of ABVD) followed by IF-RT in a dose of 30 to 36 Gy. The increasing efficacy of chemotherapy and late toxic effects of wide-field RT justify the careful testing of the new involved-node RT principle in the combined-modality approach. The identification of the unfavorable stage I/II or intermediate stage subset of patients based on the EORTC/GHSG clinical pre-treatment prognostic criteria is still valid. The prediction regarding the individual patient is not very accurate, however. For the purpose of tailoring treatment to the individual patient we need more accurate measures, preferably predictive factors that may tell us how the individual patient should be treated. The result of an early FDG-PET scan may well become the major new treatment-related guidance for an individually tailored treatment approach.

References

[1] Rosenberg SA. Report of the committee on the staging of Hodgkin's Disease. Cancer Res 1966;26:1310.

[2] Lister TA, Crowther D, Sutcliffe SB, et al. Report of a committee convened to discuss the evaluation and staging of patients with Hodgkin's disease: Cotswolds meeting. J Clin Oncol 1989;7(11):1630–6.

[3] Diehl V, Thomas RK, Re D. Part II: Hodgkin's lymphoma—diagnosis and treatment. Lancet Oncol 2004;5(1):19–26.

[4] Specht L, Hasenclever D, et al. Prognostic factors. In: Hoppe RT, Armitage JO, Diehl V, editors. Hodgkin's disease. Philadelphia: Lippincott Williams & Wilkins; 2007. p. 152–69.

[5] Gisselbrecht C, Mounier N, Andre M, et al. How to define intermediate stage in Hodgkin's lymphoma? Eur J Haematol Suppl 2005;(66):111–4.

[6] Diehl V, Franklin J, Pfreundschuh M, et al. Standard and increased-dose BEACOPP chemotherapy compared with COPP-ABVD for advanced Hodgkin's disease. N Engl J Med 2003;348(24):2386–95.

[7] Horning SJ, Hoppe RT, Breslin S, et al. Stanford V and radiotherapy for locally extensive and advanced Hodgkin's disease: mature results of a prospective clinical trial. J Clin Oncol 2002;20(3):630–7.

[8] Adams MJ, Lipsitz SR, Colan SD, et al. Cardiovascular status in long-term survivors of Hodgkin's disease treated with chest radiotherapy. J Clin Oncol 2004;22(15):3139–48.

[9] Aleman BM, van den Belt-Dusebout AW, Klokman WJ, et al. Long-term cause-specific mortality of patients treated for Hodgkin's disease. J Clin Oncol 2003;21(18):3431–9.

[10] Franklin J, Paus M, Wolf J, et al. Chemotherapy, radiotherapy and combined modality for Hodgkin's disease, with emphasis on second cancer risk. Cochrane Database Syst Rev 2005; Issue 4. Art. No.: CD003187. DOI: 10.1002/14651858. CD003187. pub 2.

[11] Franklin J, Pluetschow A, Paus M, et al. Second malignancy risk associated with treatment of Hodgkin's lymphoma: meta-analysis of the randomised trials. Ann Oncol 2006;17(12): 1749–60.

[12] Hancock SL, Tucker MA, Hoppe RT. Factors affecting late mortality from heart disease after treatment of Hodgkin's disease. JAMA 1993;270(16):1949–55.

[13] Hancock SL, et al. Cardiovascular late effects after treatment of Hodgkin lymphoma. In: Hoppe RT, Armitage JO, Diehl V, editors. Hodgkin's disease. Philadelphia: Lippincott Williams & Wilkins; 2007. p. 363–74.

[14] Henry-Amar M, Hayat M, Meerwaldt JH, et al. Causes of death after therapy for early stage Hodgkin's disease entered on EORTC protocols. EORTC Lymphoma Cooperative Group. Int J Radiat Oncol Biol Phys 1990;19(5):1155–7.

[15] Henry-Amar M. Second cancer after the treatment for Hodgkin's disease: a report from the International Database on Hodgkin's Disease. Ann Oncol 1992;3(Suppl 4):117–28.

[16] Hoppe RT. Hodgkin's disease: complications of therapy and excess mortality. Ann Oncol 1997;8(Suppl 1):115–8.

[17] Ng A, Mauch PM, Hoppe RT, et al. Life expectancy in Hodgkin lymphoma. In: Hoppe RT, Armitage JO, Diehl V, editors. Hodgkin's disease. Philadelphia: Lippincott Williams & Wilkins; 2007. p. 323–38.

[18] Ng AK, Bernardo MVP, Weller E, et al. Second malignancy after Hodgkin disease treated with radiation therapy with or without chemotherapy: long-term risks and risk factors. Blood 2002;100(6):1989–96.

[19] Travis LB, Gospodarowicz M, Curtis RE, et al. Lung cancer following chemotherapy and radiotherapy for Hodgkin's disease. J Natl Cancer Inst 2002;94(3):182–92.

[20] Travis LB, Hill DA, Dores GM, et al. Breast cancer following radiotherapy and chemotherapy among young women with Hodgkin disease. JAMA 2003;290(4):465–75.

[21] van Leeuwen FE, Swerdlow AJ, Travis LB. Second cancers after treatment of Hodgkin lymphoma. In: Hoppe RT, Armitage JO, Diehl V, et al, editors. Hodgkin's disease. Philadelphia: Lippincott Williams & Wilkins; 2007. p. 339–62.

[22] Aviles A, Arevila N, Diaz Maqueo JC, et al. Late cardiac toxicity of doxorubicin, epirubicin, and mitoxantrone therapy for Hodgkin's disease in adults. Leuk Lymphoma 1993;11(3–4): 275–9.

[23] Chronowski GM, Wilder RB, Levy LB, et al. Second malignancies after chemotherapy and radiotherapy for Hodgkin disease. Am J Clin Oncol 2004;27(1):73–80.

[24] Josting A, Wiedenmann S, Franklin J, et al. Secondary myeloid leukemia and myelodysplastic syndromes in patients treated for Hodgkin's disease: a report from the German Hodgkin's Lymphoma study group. J Clin Oncol 2003;21(18):3440–6.

[25] Moser EC, Noordijk EM, van Leeuwen FE, et al. Long-term risk of cardiovascular disease after treatment for aggressive non-Hodgkin lymphoma. Blood 2006;107(7):2912–9.

[26] Swerdlow AJ, Barber JA, Horwich A, et al. Second malignancy in patients with Hodgkin's disease treated at the Royal Marsden Hospital. Br J Cancer 1997;75(1):116–23.

[27] Swerdlow AJ, Barber JA, Hudson GV, et al. Risk of second malignancy after Hodgkin's disease in a collaborative British cohort: The relation to age at treatment. J Clin Oncol 2000;18(3):498–509.

[28] van Leeuwen FE, Chorus AM, Belt-Dusebout AW, et al. Leukemia risk following Hodgkin's disease: relation to cumulative dose of alkylating agents, treatment with teniposide combinations, number of episodes of chemotherapy, and bone marrow damage. J Clin Oncol 1994;12(5):1063–73.

[29] Bhatia R, Van Heijzen K, Palmer A, et al. Longitudinal assessment of hematopoietic abnormalities after autologous hematopoietic cell transplantation for lymphoma. J Clin Oncol 2005;23(27):6699–711.

[30] Metayer C, Curtis RE, Vose J, et al. Myelodysplastic syndrome and acute myeloid leukemia after autotransplantation for lymphoma: a multicenter case-control study. Blood 2003;101(5):2015–23.

[31] Pedersen-Bjergaard J, Andersen MK, Christiansen DH. Therapy-related acute myeloid leukemia and myelodysplasia after high-dose chemotherapy and autologous stem cell transplantation. Blood 2000;95(11):3273–9.

[32] Noordijk EM, Carde P, Dupouy N, et al. Combined-modality therapy for clinical stage I or II Hodgkin's lymphoma: long-term results of the European Organisation for Research and Treatment of Cancer H7 randomized controlled trials. J Clin Oncol 2006;24(19):3128–35.

[33] Hoerni B, Orgerie MB, Eghbali H, et al. [New combination of epirubicin, bleomycin, vinblastine and prednisone (EBVP II) before radiotherapy in localized stages of Hodgkin's disease. Phase II trial in 50 patients]. Bull Cancer 1988;75(8):789–94.

[34] Diehl V, Brillant C, Engert A, et al. HD10: investigating reduction of combined modality treatment intensity in early stage Hodgkin's lymphoma. Interim analysis of a randomized trial of the German Hodgkin Study Group (GHSG). J Clin Oncol 2005;23(16S):561s.

[35] Anselmo AP, Cavalieri E, Osti FM, et al. Intermediate stage Hodgkin's disease: preliminary results on 210 patients treated with four ABVD chemotherapy cycles plus extended versus involved field radiotherapy. Anticancer Res 2004;24(6):4045–50.

[36] Diehl V, Brillant C, Engert A, et al. Recent interim analysis of the HD11 trial of the GHSG: Intensification of chemotherapy and reduction of radiation dose in early unfavourable stage Hodgkin's lymphoma. Blood 2005;106(11):240a–1a.

[37] Engert A, Schiller P, Josting A, et al. Involved-field radiotherapy is equally effective and less toxic compared with extended-field radiotherapy after four cycles of chemotherapy in patients with early-stage unfavorable Hodgkin's lymphoma: results of the HD8 trial of the German Hodgkin's Lymphoma study group. J Clin Oncol 2003;21(19):3601–8.

[38] Ferme C, Eghbali H, Hagenbeek A, et al. MOPP/ABV hybrid and irradiation in unfavorable supradiaphragmatic clinical stages I-II Hodgkin's disease: comparison of three treatment modalities. Preliminary results of the EORTC-GELA H8-U randomized trial in 995 patients. Blood 2000;96:A576.

[39] Ferme C, Divine M, Vranovsky A, et al. Four ABVD and involved-field radiotherapy in unfavourable supradiaphragmatic clinical stages (CS) I-II Hodgkin's lymphoma (HL): results of the EORTC-GELA H9-U trial. Blood 2005;106(11):240a.

[40] Meyer RM, Gospodarowicz MK, Connors JM, et al. Randomized comparison of ABVD chemotherapy with a strategy that includes radiation therapy in patients with limited-stage Hodgkin's lymphoma: National Cancer Institute of Canada Clinical Trials Group and the Eastern Cooperative Oncology Group. J Clin Oncol 2005;23(21):4634–42.

[41] Sieber M, Tesch H, Pfistner B, et al. Rapidly alternating COPP/ABV/IMEP is not superior to conventional alternating COPP/ABVD in combination with extended-field radiotherapy in intermediate-stage Hodgkin's Lymphoma: final results of the German Hodgkin's Lymphoma study group trial HD5. J Clin Oncol 2002;20(2):476–84.

[42] Bonadonna G, Zucali R, Monfardini S, et al. Combination chemotherapy of Hodgkin's disease with Adriamycin, bleomycin, vinblastine, and imidazole carboxamide versus MOPP. Cancer 1975;36(1):252–9.

[43] Canellos GP, Niedzwiecki D. Long-term follow-up of Hodgkin's disease trial. N Engl J Med 2002;346(18):1417–8.

[44] Duggan DB, Petroni GR, Johnson JL, et al. Randomized comparison of ABVD and MOPP/ABV hybrid for the treatment of advanced Hodgkin's disease: report of an intergroup trial. J Clin Oncol 2003;21(4):607–14.

[45] Le Maignan C, Desablens B, Delwail V, et al. Three cycles of Adriamycin, bleomycin, vinblastine, and dacarbazine (ABVD) or epirubicin, bleomycin, vinblastine, and methotrexate (EBVM) plus extended field radiation therapy in early and intermediate Hodgkin disease: 10-year results of a randomized trial. Blood 2004;103(1):58–66.

[46] Longo DL, Glatstein E, Duffey PL, et al. A prospective trial of radiation alone vs combination chemotherapy alone for early-stage Hodgkin's disease: implications of 25-year follow-up to current combined modality therapy. Blood 2006;108(11):33a.

[47] Press OW, LeBlanc M, Lichter AS, et al. Phase III randomized intergroup trial of subtotal lymphoid irradiation versus doxorubicin, vinblastine, and subtotal lymphoid irradiation for stage IA to IIA Hodgkin's disease. J Clin Oncol 2001;19(22):4238–44.

[48] Straus DJ, Portlock CS, Qin J, et al. Results of a prospective randomized clinical trial of doxorubicin, bleomycin, vinblastine, and dacarbazine (ABVD) followed by radiation therapy (RT) versus ABVD alone for stages I, II, and IIIA nonbulky Hodgkin disease. Blood 2004;104(12):3483–9.

[49] Hasenclever D, Diehl V. A prognostic score for advanced Hodgkin's disease. International prognostic factors project on advanced Hodgkin's Disease. N Engl J Med 1998;339(21):1506–14.

[50] Carde P, Koscielny S, Franklin J, et al. Early response to chemotherapy: a surrogate for final outcome of Hodgkin's disease patients that should influence initial treatment length and intensity? Ann Oncol 2002;13:86–91.

[51] Aleman BM, Raemaekers JM, Tirelli U, et al. Involved-field radiotherapy for advanced Hodgkin's lymphoma. N Engl J Med 2003;348(24):2396–406.

[52] Carde P. The chemotherapy/radiation balance in advanced Hodgkin's lymphoma: overweight which side? J Clin Oncol 2005;23(36):9058–62.

[53] Connors JM. State-of-the-art therapeutics: Hodgkin's lymphoma. J Clin Oncol 2005;23(26):6400–8.

[54] DeVita VT Jr. Hodgkin's disease—clinical trials and travails. N Engl J Med 2003;348(24): 2375–6.

[55] Diehl V, Schiller P, Engert A, et al. Results of the 3rd interim analysis of the HD12 trial of the GHSG: 8 courses of escalated BEACOPP with or without additive radiotherapy for advanced stage Hodgkin's lymphoma. Blood 2003;102(11):27a–8a.

[56] Diehl V. Chemotherapy or combined modality treatment: the optimal treatment for Hodgkin's disease. J Clin Oncol 2004;22(1):15–8.

[57] Ferme C, Sebban C, Hennequin C, et al. Comparison of chemotherapy to radiotherapy as consolidation of complete or good partial response after six cycles of chemotherapy for patients with advanced Hodgkin's disease: results of the Groupe d'Etudes des Lymphomes de l'Adulte H89 trial. Blood 2000;95(7):2246–52.

[58] Laskar S, Gupta T, Vimal S, et al. Consolidation radiation after complete remission in Hodgkin's disease following six cycles of doxorubicin, bleomycin, vinblastine, and dacarbazine chemotherapy: is there a need? J Clin Oncol 2004;22(1):62–8.

[59] Loeffler M, Brosteanu O, Hasenclever D, et al. Meta-analysis of chemotherapy versus combined modality treatment trials in Hodgkin's disease. International Database on Hodgkin's Disease overview study group. J Clin Oncol 1998;16(3):818–29.

[60] Longo DL. Radiation therapy in the treatment of Hodgkin's disease—do you see what I see? J Natl Cancer Inst 2003;95(13):928–9.

[61] van der Maazen RW, Raemaekers JM. Chemotherapy and radiotherapy in Hodgkin's lymphoma: joining in or splitting up? Curr Opin Oncol 2006;18(6):660–6.

[62] Yahalom J. Don't throw out the baby with the bathwater: on optimizing cure and reducing toxicity in Hodgkin's lymphoma. J Clin Oncol 2006;24(4):544–8.

[63] Aleman BM, Raemaekers JM, Tomisic R, et al. Involved-field radiotherapy for patients in partial remission after chemotherapy for advanced Hodgkin's lymphoma. Int J Radiat Oncol Biol Phys 2007;67(1):19–30.

[64] Franklin J, Paulus U, Lieberz D, et al. Is the international prognostic score for advanced stage Hodgkin's disease applicable to early stage patients? German Hodgkin Lymphoma study group. Ann Oncol 2000;11(5):617–23.

[65] Bohlius J, Haverkamp H, Diehl V, et al. Identification of prognostic factors in early unfavorable stage Hodgkin's lymphoma (HL): an individual patient data meta-analysis. Blood 2006;108(11):700a.

[66] Klimm B, Eich H, Haverkamp H, et al. Poorer outcome of elderly patients treated with extended-field radiotherapy compared with involved-field radiotherapy after chemotherapy for Hodgkin's lymphoma: an analysis from the German Hodgkin Study Group. Ann Oncol 2007;18(2):357–63.

[67] Advani R, Maeda L, Hoppe RT, et al. Assessment of favorable (F) versus unfavorable (U) early stage Hodgkin's disease (HD): the Stanford V + radiotherapy (RT) experience. Blood 2005;106(11):548a.

[68] Tartas NE, Zerga M, Santos MI, et al. International prognostic score (IPS) is not useful in stages I-II Hodgkin's lymphoma (HL)—an experience of the Buenos Aires Leukemia Group (BALG). Blood 2006;108(Suppl part 2):246b.

[69] Hutchings M, Loft A, Hansen M, et al. FDG-PET after two cycles of chemotherapy predicts treatment failure and progression-free survival in Hodgkin lymphoma. Blood 2006;107(1):52–9.

[70] Gallamini A, Rigacci L, Merli F, et al. The predictive value of positron emission tomography scanning performed after two courses of standard therapy on treatment outcome in advanced stage Hodgkin's disease. Haematologica 2006;91(4):475–81.

[71] Kostakoglu L, Coleman M, Leonard JP, et al. PET predicts prognosis after 1 cycle of chemotherapy in aggressive lymphoma and Hodgkin's disease. J Nucl Med 2002;43(8): 1018–27.

[72] Zinzani PL, Tani M, Fanti S, et al. Early positron emission tomography (PET) restaging: a predictive final response in Hodgkin's disease patients. Ann Oncol 2006;17(8):1296–300.

[73] Cheson BD, Pfistner B, Juweid ME, et al. Revised response criteria for malignant lymphoma. J Clin Oncol 2007;25(5):579–86.

[74] Girinsky T, van der Maazen R, Specht L, et al. Involved-node radiotherapy (INRT) in patients with early Hodgkin lymphoma: concepts and guidelines. Radiother Oncol 2006;79(3): 270–7.

New Strategies for the Treatment of Advanced-Stage Hodgkin's Lymphoma

Volker Diehl, MD[a],*, Andreas Engert, MD[b], Daniel Re, MD[b]

[a]Department of Internal Medicine I, Haus Lebenswert, University Hospital of Cologne, Kerpenerstr. 62, 50931 Cologne, Germany
[b]Department of Internal Medicine I, University Hospital of Cologne, Kerpenerstr. 62, 50931 Cologne, Germany

Hodgkin's lymphoma (HL) is one of the most curable cancers of adulthood. In localized stages of the disease more than 95% of patients can be cured with modern treatment strategies. In advanced stages, composed of stages IIB with large mediastinal tumors and all stages III and IV according to the Ann Arbor classification, more than 85% of patients experience long-term tumor-free survival. In the current cohorts of HL survivors after 15 years more individuals have died of adverse sequelae of treatment than of Hodgkin's-related causes of death. Current intentions for improvement therefore aim for preserving the high cure rates while reducing the acute and long-term toxicities. The definition of advanced HL varies considerably between different study groups and is summarized in Table 1.

EARLY AND ADVANCED HODGKIN'S LYMPHOMA

In North America, in contrast to the original National Cancer Institute (NCI) study, most groups and clinical centers have included patients who had bulky stage I and II or IIB disease under the heading of "advanced" Hodgkin's lymphoma. This diversity of risk allocation resulting also in different treatment strategies made the comparison of treatment results difficult. Furthermore, there was a considerable heterogeneity concerning response and outcome criteria.

The recent International Harmonization Project attempts to standardize response assessment and outcome measurements and will facilitate comparison of results in clinical trials [1].

Staging laparotomy as a routine staging technique has become obsolete. We now rely on more sensitive anatomic and functional imaging techniques to

*Corresponding author. E-mail address: v.diehl@uni-koeln.de (V. Diehl).

0889-8588/07/$ – see front matter
doi:10.1016/j.hoc.2007.07.004
© 2007 Elsevier Inc. All rights reserved.
hemonc.theclinics.com

Table 1
Definition of treatment groups according to the European Organization for Research and Treatment of Cancer/Groupe d'Etude des Lymphomes de l'Adulte, German Hodgkin's Lymphoma Study Group, and National Cancer Institute of Canada/Eastern Cooperative Oncology Group

Treatment group	EORTC/GELA	GHSG	NCIC/ECOG
Early stage favorable	CS I–II without risk factors (supradiaphragmatic)	CS I–II without risk factors	Standard risk group: favorable CS I–II (without risk factors)
Early stage unfavorable (intermediate)	CS I–II with ≥1 risk factor (supradiaphragmatic)	CS I, CSIIA ≥1 risk factors; CS IIB with C/D but without A/B	Standard risk group: unfavorable CS I–II (at least one risk factor)
Advanced stage	CS III–IV	CS IIB with A/B; CS III–IV	High risk group: CS I or II with bulky disease; intraabdominal disease; CS III, IV
Risk factors (RF)	A. Large mediastinal mass B. Age ≥50 years C. Elevated ESR^a D. ≥4 involved regions	A. Large mediastinal mass B. Extranodal disease C. Elevated ESR^a D. ≥3 involved areas	A. ≥40 years B. Not NLPHL or NS histology C. ESR ≥50 mm/h D. ≥4 involved nodal regions

Abbreviations: ECOG, Eastern Cooperative Oncology Group; EORTC, European Organization for Research and Treatment of Cancer; GELA, Groupe d'Etude des Lymphomes de l'Adulte; GHSG, German Hodgkin Study Group; NCIC, National Cancer Institute of Canada; NLPHL, nodular lymphocyte predominance; NS, nodular sclerosis.
^{a}Erythrocyte sedimentation rate (≥50 mm/h without or ≥30 mm/h with B symptoms).

localize tumorous lesions to assign patients to an exact Ann Arbor stage, with complementary clinical- biologic risk groups.

With the determination of clinical and biologic risk factors, described in the International Prognostic Score (IPS), it is possible to allocate patients at diagnosis to certain risk groups, facilitating risk-adapted therapy planning (Table 2).

With more sensitive morphologic radiographic imaging techniques and functional imaging with FDG-positron emission tomography (PET) it becomes possible to assess early treatment response, thus enabling the doctor to tailor therapy according to the individual necessity of escalating or reducing treatment intensity, providing the chance for an individualized, risk- and response-adapted treatment strategy in hopes of sparing the patient unnecessary toxicity while pertaining the highest efficacy [1].

Table 2
International prognostic factors for Hodgkin's lymphoma

No. of factors[a]	Population (%)	Estimated freedom from disease progression at 5 years (%)
0	7	84
1	22	77
2	29	67
3	23	60
4	12	51
5+	7	42

[a]Factors: Stage IV; male sex; age $\geq$45 years; hemoglobin <10.5 G/dL; WBC$\geq$15,000/μL; lymphocytes <8% or <600/μL; albumin <4 G/dL.

Data from Hasenclever D, Diehl V. A prognostic score for advanced Hodgkin's disease. International Prognostic Factors Project on Advanced Hodgkin's Disease. N Engl J Med 1998;339(21):1506–14.

PROGNOSTIC FACTORS IN ADVANCED-STAGE HODGKIN'S LYMPHOMA

When aiming at drug or time intensification of therapy it is mandatory to precisely define the group of patients who might benefit from dose escalation despite a higher risk for toxicity, and to spare the cohort that might suffice with the standard treatment. Unlike non-Hodgkin's lymphomas or acute and chronic leukemias no robust molecular, molecular-genetic, immunocytologic, or other biologic risk or prognostic factors exist yet in HL. The IPS, resulting from an international project involving more than 5,000 patients, led by Hasenclever and Diehl [2], identified prognostic factors in advanced Hodgkin's lymphoma. Seven factors were recognized—stage IV, male sex, age, hemoglobin, white blood count, lymphocyte count, albumin—each of which contributed about a 7% reduction in freedom from progression at 5 years (Table 3). When five to seven adverse factors were present, one of which included age older than 45 years, freedom from progression at 5 years fell to 45% [3]. This subgroup was small and constituted only 7% of the total patient population, however, indicating that large numbers of patients recruited to randomized trials would be necessary to investigate new therapeutic strategies in this cohort of patients.

FIRST- AND SECOND-GENERATION CHEMOTHERAPY: MOPP AND ABVD

Despite the excellent results achieved with mechlorethamine, vincristine (Oncovin), procarbazine, and prednisone (MOPP) [4], there was the need to obtain equivalent or improved results with less gastrointestinal and neurologic toxicity. In 1975 Bonadonna and colleagues [5] introduced the novel ABVD [Adriamycin (doxorubicin), bleomycin, vinblastine, and dacarbazine] regimen for patients who had failed MOPP chemotherapy. ABVD was specifically developed for MOPP resistance, incorporating four different individually effective compounds. Results of selected trials are summarized in Table 4 [6].

Table 3
Seven-year results of German Hodgkin Lymphoma Study Group HD9 trial according to International Prognostic Score

	IPS = 0–1, N = 306		IPS = 2–3, N = 465		IPS≥4, N = 169	
	FFTF	OS	FFTF	OS	FFTF	OS
COPP/ABVD	78%	89%	64%	78%	59%	66%
BEACOPP	83%	91%	73%	84%	74%	79%
BEACOPP-escalated	91%	93%	83%	90%	81%	83%
P	0.023	0.53	0.0017	0.042	0.23	0.6

Abbreviations: ABVD, doxorubicin, bleomycin, vinblastine, and dacarbazine; BEACOPP, bleomycin, etoposide, adriamycin, cyclophosphamide, vincristin, procarbazine, prednisone; COPP, cyclophosphamide, vincristine, procarbazine, and prednisone; FFTF, freedom from treatment failure; GHSG, German Hodgkin Study Group; IPS, International Prognostic Score; OS, overall survival.
   Data from Hasenclever D, Diehl V. A prognostic score for advanced Hodgkin's disease. International Prognostic Factors Project on Advanced Hodgkin's Disease. N Engl J Med 1998;339(21):1506–14.

ALTERNATING MOPP/ABVD AND HYBRID MOPP/ABV REGIMEN (THIRD GENERATION)

Based on data originating from pilot studies from Bonadonna's group, in which cycles of MOPP and ABVD were alternated in patients who had stage IV disease, the CALGB compared in a three-arm trial the relative efficacy and toxicity of 6 to 8 cycles of MOPP, 6 to 8 cycles of ABVD, and 12 cycles of

Table 4
Randomized trials with ABVD chemotherapy

Group and treatment	No. of cycles	RT	No. of patients	Stage	% FFP (P)	% FFS (P)	% OS (P)	Time analyzed (y)
Milan [5]	6	IF	76	IIB, III, IV				10
ABVD	6				63		54	
MOPP	6				50		39 (NS)	
					(NS)			
Milan [6]		STLI	232	IIB, III				7
ABVD	6				81		77	
MOPP	6				63		68	
					(<.002)		(<.03)	
CALGB [7]	—		361	III, IV prior RT				5
ABVD	6–8					61	73	
MOPP	6–8					50	66	
MOPP/ABVD	12					65	75	
						(.03)	(NS)	

Abbreviations: CALBG, Cancer and Leukemia Group B; FFP, freedom from progression; FFS, failure-free survival; IF, involved field; NS, not significant; OS, overall survival; STLI, subtotal lymphoid irradiation; RT, radiotherapy.

Table 5

Efficacy and toxicity of MOPP ABV of ABVD

Group and treatment	No. of cycles	No. of patients	Stage	% FFS (P)	% OS (P)	Time analyzed (y)	Toxicity
NCI-Canada [11]		301	III, IV prior RT			5	
Alternating MOPP/ABVD ± RT[c]	8–12			67	83		More febrile neutropenia and mucositis with MOPP/ABV
Hybrid MOPP/ABV ± RT[c]	8–12			71 (NS)	81 (NS)		No difference in toxic deaths or second malignancy
Milan [8]		427	I–IIB[b], III, IV prior RT			10	
Alternating MOPP/ABVD ± RT[c]	6–8			67[d]	74		6% incidence of second malignancy in all treated patients
Hybrid MOPP-ABVD ± RT[c]	6–8			65 (NS)	72 (NS)		
ECOG [9]		737	III, IV prior RT			8	
Hybrid MOPP-ABV	8–12			64	79		More neutropenia and pulmonary toxicity with hybrid; more leukemia/MDS with sequential
Sequential MOPP→ABVD	9–11			54 (.01)	71 (.02)		
CALGB [12]		856	III, IV prior RT			5	
Hybrid MOPP/ABV	8–10			66	81		More neutropenia and pulmonary toxicity with hybrid; more leukemia/MDS with sequential
ABVD	8–10			63 (NS)	82 (NS)		

Abbreviations: CALGB, Cancer and Leukemia Group B; ECOG, Eastern Cooperative Oncology Group; FFS, failure free survival; MDS, myelodysplastic syndrome; NS, not significant; OS, overall survival; RT, radiation therapy.
[a]RT given for residual disease.
[b]IIA bulky also included.
[c]RT given for bulky disease.
[d]Freedom from progression.

MOPP alternating with ABVD in patients who had advanced Hodgkin's lymphoma (see Table 4; Table 5) [7–9].

A total of 361 eligible patients were randomized to MOPP (n = 123), ABVD (n = 115), or alternating (n = 123) therapy. The 10-year failure-free survival rates were 38% for MOPP, 55% for ABVD, and 50% for MOPP/ABVD, P = .02. There was a trend for superior overall survival for ABVD (68%) or MOPP/ABVD (65%) compared with MOPP alone (58%, P = .15).

In 1985, Klimo and Connors [10] for the first time reported a study in previously untreated patients who had stage IIEA, III, and IV disease in which they tested a MOPP-ABV hybrid, with MOPP given on days 1 to 7 and ABV on day 8. Doxorubicin was increased from 25 to 35 mg/m^2 and dacarbazine was omitted. Prednisone was given for 14 days. Involved-field irradiation was given to partial responders. Some 88% achieved a complete remission and overall survival was 90% at 4 years.

Based on these encouraging data, the National Cancer Institute of Canada embarked on a trial comparing MOPP-ABV hybrid with alternating MOPP/ABVD in patients who had IIIB or IV HL or those who had previously received wide-field irradiation (see Table 5) [11]. Responding patients received a minimum of eight cycles of chemotherapy and those who had residual disease in a localized region received irradiation between the sixth and seventh cycles. The overall survival rates at 5 years in the 301 randomized patients were similar (81% MOPP-ABV hybrid, 83% alternating MOPP/ABVD; P = .74). Failure-free survivals were also similar (71% MOPP-ABV hybrid, 67% alternating MOPP/ABVD; P = .87). The hybrid regimen proved to be more toxic with a higher incidence of febrile neutropenia and stomatitis.

The promising data of a series of North American and European trials with the hybrid regimen MOPP/ABV led investigators in North America to launch an intergroup trial comparing ABVD with MOPP/ABV. A total of 856 patients who had stage III or IV HL or relapses following irradiation were randomized to a minimum of eight cycles of chemotherapy [12]. There was no difference in failure-free survival for ABVD (63%) or MOPP-ABV (66%), P = .42 at 5 years.

Although no difference in overall survival was seen (82% for ABVD and 81% for MOPP-ABV; P = .82), hematologic and pulmonary toxicities were significantly greater with hybrid treatment (P = .06 and .001). This finding led the Data and Safety Monitoring Board to stop the study prematurely because of excess of treatment-related deaths and second malignancies with the hybrid regimen.

In conclusion, neither (C)MOPP, the alternating MOPP and ABVD, nor the hybrid setting was superior to the ABVD regimen alone, establishing ABVD, at least in North America, as the treatment of choice for advanced Hodgkin's lymphoma and making ABVD the regimen to which new treatments need to be compared.

TIME- AND DOSE-INTENSIFIED REGIMEN (FOURTH GENERATION)

New dose- and time-intensified or time-dense regimens, supported by hematopoietic growth factors, facilitate the delivery of higher and more prolonged concentrations of cytotoxic drugs, ensuring more effective tumor control. Recent data on studies with now more than 9 years of median observation time support the assumption that these strategies also offer an improved long-term survival. Whether there is an overall benefit compared with treatment-related complications, however, awaits even longer-term follow-up of more than 10 to 15 years from recent and current clinical trials.

THE STANFORD V PROGRAM

The Stanford group took another approach to the concern for late toxicity in the management of HL [13]. They devised Stanford V, a seven-drug regimen that includes weekly treatment given over 12 weeks for patients who have locally extensive or advanced HL. Compared with ABVD or hybrid regimens Stanford V maintains or increases the dose intensity of individual drugs but reduces the cumulative doses of doxorubicin, mechlorethamine, and bleomycin compared with the doses in MOPP/ABV(D) or ABVD alone and omits procarbazine. An important feature of Stanford V is the use of consolidative radiotherapy (36 Gy) to sites of disease 5 cm or greater at diagnosis and macroscopic splenic involvement. Mature results from a phase II study of 162 patients at Stanford report a freedom from progression (FFP) of 89% and overall survival (OS) of 96%, with a median follow-up of 5.4 years. The 71% of patients who had zero to two risk factors according to the IPS had an FFP of 94%, compared with 75% for patients who had three or more risk factors.

The OS for this high-risk group was still greater than 90% because of effective salvage therapy. The main toxicities were neutropenia and constipation. No cases of bleomycin toxicity or radiation pneumonitis were observed. In addition no cases of secondary myelodysplasia (MDS)/leukemia or lymphoma have been reported to date [14].

Two recent randomized trials compare Stanford V to ABVD in patients who have advanced disease. The ECOG 2496 intergroup trial compared the Stanford V program (chemotherapy plus radiation as defined above) with ABVD plus radiation for bulky mediastinal disease and an ongoing United Kingdom study in which Stanford V plus radiation is compared with ABVD plus radiation (a follow-up to the pilot study noted above). Mature results from both these trials are awaited to evaluate the long-term effects for cure and for complications.

Recently, another group from Italy (Intergruppo Italiano Linfomi) compared ABVD to a modified Stanford V program and a multiagent chemotherapy regimen consisting of mechlorethamine, vincristine, procarbazine, prednisone, epidoxorubicin, bleomycin, vinblastine, lomustine, doxorubicin, and vindesine (MOPPEBVCAD) [15]. In this study, the 5-year FFS and progression free survival for the modified Stanford V arm was inferior to the other two regimens, with no differences in overall survival. The interpretation of these results is confounded for several reasons. First, the response evaluation, which determined whether patients continued on the study arm, was completed at different times: after 8 weeks of Stanford V chemotherapy, 16 weeks for ABVD, and 24 weeks for MOPPEBVCAD. Second, the modifications to radiotherapy were substantial, including a limit on the number of treated sites, a different definition of bulk, and a delay in initiating radiotherapy to a median of 6 weeks. The proportion of patients who received consolidative irradiation was substantially less than in the series reported from Stanford and ECOG (66% versus 90%). It is difficult to compare the outcomes of these different studies because patient selection and prognostic variables varied. One possible explanation for the different outcomes in the abbreviated chemotherapy programs is the variable use of radiotherapy as a consolidative therapy.

THE BEACOPP REGIMEN

Drug delivery may be intensified by increasing individual drug dose, shortening the interval between treatments, or both. The German Hodgkin Study Group (GHSG) has completed a series of studies that address these issues of dose intensity. A mathematical model of tumor growth and chemotherapy effects fitted to the data from 705 patients treated by the GHSG served as the basis for these studies [3]. This model predicted that moderate dose escalation would improve failure-free survival by 10% to 15% at 5 years. The BEACOPP regimen (Table 6) was devised to serve as a standard combination for dose escalation.

With the design of standard and escalated BEACOPP in place, in 1992 the GHSG started a three-arm trial (HD9) in which these combinations were prospectively tested together with COPP/ABVD in advanced HL [16]. All three arms of this randomized trial included 30-Gy consolidative radiotherapy for initially bulky (>5 cm) or residual disease, which was administered to 61% to 70% of the patients. The pooled BEACOPP arms were superior to COPP/ABVD regarding progression rate and freedom from treatment failure in the interim analyses, and the COPP/ABVD arm was closed early to further accrual. In the most recent report, which included 1186 evaluable patients who had median follow-up of 7 years, the freedom from treatment failure (FFTF) was 67% in the COPP/ABVD group, 75% in the BEACOPP group, and 85% in the increased-dose BEACOPP.

The induction failure rates were 25%, 12%, and 4%. Overall survival rates were 79%, 84%, and 90% for COPP/ABVD, BEACOPP, and the increased-dose BEACOPP, respectively, with the difference between COPP/ABVD and increased-dose BEACOPP being significant ($P < .002$). Although the two BEACOPP regimens were superior to COPP/ABVD in all prognostic groups, the most pronounced differences were in the poor-risk group of patients who had four to seven adverse factors according to the IPS (Table 7). As expected, the escalated BEACOPP was associated with greater hematologic

Table 6
Etoposide-containing combination chemotherapy

Drug combination	Dose (mg/m^2)	Route	Schedule (d)	RT	Cycle/ length (d)
Alkylating agent-containing					
BEACOPP (escalated BEACOPP)				Bulky, residual	21
Bleomycin	10	IV	8		
Etoposide	100 (200)	IV	1–3		
Adriamycin (doxorubicin)	25 (35)	IV	1		
Cyclophosphamide	650 (1250)	IV	1		
Oncovin (vincristine)	1.4[a]	IV	8		
Procarbazine	100	PO	1–7		
Prednisone	40	PO	1–14		
G-CSF	≃(+)	SQ	8+		
BEACOPP-14				Bulky, residual	14
Cyclophosphamide	650	IV	1		
Adriamycin	25	IV	1		
Etoposide	100	IV	1–3		
Procarbazine	100	PO	1–7		
Prednisone	80	PO	1–7		
Vincristine	1.4 (max. 2)	IV	8		
Bleomycin	10	IV	8		
G-CSF		SC	from day 8		
Stanford V				Bulky	12 wk
Mechlorethamine	6	IV	Wk 1, 5, 9		
Adriamycin (doxorubicin)	25	IV	Wk 1, 3, 5, 9, 11		
Vinblastine	6	IV	Wk 1, 3, 5, 9, 11		
Vincristine	1.4[a]	IV	Wk 2, 4, 6, 8, 10, 12		
Bleomycin	5	IV	Wk 2, 4, 6, 8, 10, 12		
Etoposide	60 × 2	IV	Wk 3, 7, 11		
Prednisone	40	PO	Wk 1–10 qod		
G-CSF			Dose reduction or delay		
OEPA/COPP[b]				IF	28
Oncovin (vincristine)	1.5[a]	IV	1, 8, 15		
Etoposide	125	IV	3–6		
Prednisone	60	PO	1–15		
Adriamycin (doxorubicin)	40	IV	1, 15		
ChlVPP/EVA				—	28
Chlorambucil	10 total	PO	1–7		
Vinblastine	10 total	IV	1		
Procarbazine	150 total	PO	1–7		
Prednisolone	50 total	PO	1–7		
Etoposide	200	IV	8		
Vincristine	2 total	IV	8		
Adriamycin (doxorubicin)	50	IV	8		

(continued on next page)

Table 6
(continued)

Drug combination	Dose (mg/m²)	Route	Schedule (d)	RT	Cycle/ length (d)
ChlVPP/PABLOE				Bulky	50
Chlorambucil	6	PO	1–14		
Vinblastine	6	IV	1, 8		
Procarbazine	100	PO	1–14, 29–43		
Prednisolone	30	PO	1–14		
Adriamycin (doxorubicin)	40	IV	29		
Bleomycin	10	IV	29, 36		
Vincristine	1.4ᵃ	IV	29, 36		
Etoposide	200	PO	30–32		
VAPEC-B				Bulky, residual	11 wk
Vincristine	1.4ᵃ	IV	Wk 2, 4, 6, 8, 10		
Adriamycin (doxorubicin)	35	IV	Wk 1, 3, 5, 7, 9, 11		
Prednisolone	50	PO	Wk 1–6		
Etoposide	75–100 × 5	PO	Wk 3, 7, 11		
Cyclophosphamide	350	IV	Wk 1, 5, 9		
Bleomycin	10	IV	Wk 2, 4, 6, 8, 10		
Non–alkylating agent–containing					
EVA				Bulky, residual	28
Etoposide	100	IV	1–3		
Vinblastine	6	IV	1		
Adriamycin (doxorubicin)	50	IV	1		
VEPA				IF	28
Vinblastine	6	IV	1, 15		
Etoposide	200	IV	1, 15		
Prednisone	40	PO	1–14		
Adriamycin (doxorubicin)	25	IV	1,15		

Abbreviations: G-CSF, granulocyte colony-stimulating factor; IF, involved field; IV, intravenous; PO, oral; SQ, subcutaneous.
ᵃVincristine dose capped at 2 mg.
ᵇTwo cycles of OEPA followed by two to four cycles COPP.

toxicity, including red blood cell and platelet transfusions, neutropenia, and time in hospital, although patients were generally treated in the outpatient setting. The high cumulative doses of alkylating agents and etoposide predicted that sterility and an increased risk for leukemia/MDS would complicate the use of BEACOPP. After 7 years median observation time the cumulative incidence of all secondary neoplasias were 5.2%, 6.8%, and 6.0%, respectively, for the arms COPP/ABVD, standard BEACOPP, and escalated BEACOPP, whereas the leukemia/MDS rate was 0.5% for COPP/ABVD and 2.9% for

Table 7
Design of major randomized trials in adult stage III–IV Hodgkin's lymphoma testing the value of combined modality therapy versus chemotherapy alone

	Dates	No. patients	Chemotherapy	Radiotherapy
SWOG 7808	1978–1988	590	MOP-BAP × 6	IF 20 Gy nodal 10–15 other
GHSG HD3	1984–1988	288	COPP/ABVD × 6	IF 20 Gy nodal
GELA H89	1989–1996	559	MOPP/ABVD × 6 ABVPP × 6	STNI/TNI 30 Gy nodal 5–10 Gy boosts
EORTC 20884	1989–2000	739	MOPP-ABV × 6-8	IF 24 Gy nodal 16–24 other

Abbreviations: ABV, doxorubicin, bleomycin, vinblastine; ABVD, doxorubicin, bleomycin, vinblastine, and dacarbazine; ABVPP, doxorubicin, bleomycin, vinblastine, procarbazine, and prednisone; COPP, cyclophosphamide, vincristine, procarbazine, and prednisone; EORTC, European Organization for the Research and Treatment of Cancer; GELA, Group d'Etude des Lymphome d'Adulte; GHSG, German Hodgkin Study Group; IF, involved-field irradiation; MOP-BAP, nitrogen mustard, vincristine, procarbazine, bleomycin, doxorubicin, and prednisone; STNI/TNI, subtotal/total nodal irradiation; SWOG, Southwest Oncology Group.

escalated BEACOPP. The 11% superiority in OS of increased BEACOPP over the usual standard COPP/ABVD in the recent analysis after 10 years has stabilized and offers hope for higher long-term cure rates.

The next trial of the GHSG, HD12, assigned patients to treatment with eight cycles of escalated BEACOPP or four cycles of escalated BEACOPP plus four cycles of baseline BEACOPP. Following chemotherapy, patients were randomized to receive 30 Gy irradiation to initial bulky or residual disease, versus no further therapy. After a median follow-up of 2 years with 908 evaluable patients, FFTF and OS for the whole cohort were 88% and 94%, respectively. For the group getting four escalated BEACOPP + four baseline BEACOPP, FFTF was 88% and OS 94%, respectively; for the patient cohort getting eight escalated BEACOPP, FFTF was 90% and OS 96%. There were no statistical differences between the two different treatment arms for either outcome measure and the toxicity profile was similar to that seen in the HD9 trial.

Experience with the toxicity of the escalated BEACOPP regimen, especially the risk for leukemia/MDS, next led the GHSG to develop a BEACOPP variant in which the drug dosage and timing of administration was calculated to achieve the same efficacy with reduced toxicity, according to the dose model of Hasenclever. The result was a time-intensified BEACOPP baseline regimen given in 14-day intervals and facilitated by the use of granulocyte colony stimulating factor (G-CSF), BEACOPP-14 (see Table 6).

THE BEACOPP-14 REGIMEN

In a multicenter pilot study, the GHSG tested the feasibility, toxicity, and efficacy of BEACOPP-14 in 99 patients who had advanced disease [17]. A total of 91% of the patients completed all eight cycles, 77% of courses were completed within 16 days, and 94% of courses within 22 days. Some 70% of the patients received consolidative irradiation; 94% of patients achieved a complete remission (CR) and only 4 patients had progressive disease. The OS and FFTF at 5 years were 95% and 90%, respectively. The acute hematologic toxicity was moderate, intermediate between that of the escalated and the baseline BEACOPP-21 regimens, with 80% of patients experiencing World Health Organization (WHO) grade 3 or 4 leukopenia, 27% thrombocytopenia, and 70% anemia. There were 13% of patients who had documented WHO grade III infection.

Based on the results of this pilot study, BEACOPP-14 was introduced in the HD15 trial. In this three-arm trial, patients are treated with eight cycles of escalated BEACOPP, six cycles of escalated BEACOPP, or eight cycles of BEACOPP-14. Patients who achieve only a partial response receive radiotherapy to PET-positive residual disease.

Other cooperative clinical trial groups have also tested BEACOPP for advanced-stage Hodgkin's lymphoma. The European Organization for Research and treatment of Cancer/Groupe d'Etude des Lymphomes de l'Adulte (EORTC/GELA) joined with the Nordic group, NCI Canada, British National Lymphoma Investigation, Australian Lymphoma Group, and two Spanish groups to initiate the 20012 trial. This trial compares eight cycles of ABVD to four escalated BEACOPP followed by four standard BEACOPP. An ongoing Italian trial compares the same two chemotherapy programs with MEC chemotherapy.

OTHER CHEMOTHERAPY REGIMENS

Groups in Boston and the United Kingdom initially tested the EVA [etoposide, vinblastine, Adriamycin (doxorubicin)] regimen in disease recurrent after MOPP or mechlorethamine, vinblastine, procarbazine, and prednisone (MVPP) (see Table 3) [18]. The Yale group conducted a study in 26 previously untreated patients who had locally extensive symptomatic or advanced HL in which six cycles of EVA were followed by low-dose involved-field radiotherapy in responding patients [19]. The estimated 2-year failure-free survival in these patients was just 44%. Results with EVA plus radiotherapy were also reported by the Boston group in bulky stage II (n = 20) and advanced (n = 20) disease [20]. With a median follow-up of 111 months, the failure-free survival was 57%. A group of 66 pediatric patients who had unfavorable or advanced HL was enrolled in a collaborative study of VEPA [vinblastine, etoposide, prednisone, Adriamycin (doxorubicin)] and low-dose consolidative radiotherapy conducted at Stanford University, Dana-Farber Cancer Institute, and St. Jude Children's Research Hospital [21]. This study was stopped when, with 15 months of follow-up, a projected failure-free survival of 66% was observed, a result inferior to historical controls.

These data suggest that etoposide-based regimens that do not include alkylating agents may be inferior treatments for advanced HL. That all three components in the EVA-type regimens are natural products that share the multidrug resistance phenotype may provide an explanation for these unexpected results. In contrast, chemotherapy combinations that incorporate etoposide and alkylating agents [BEACOPP, OEPA (Oncovin, etoposide, prednisone, Adriamycin)-COPP, ChlVPP/EVA, and Stanford V] have been associated with excellent results.

When comparing outcomes of clinical trials between different study groups patient selection variables (prognostic factors) seem to be of greater significance than outlay and design of the study and the drug regimen used. Randomized trials continue to be the only reliable method of determining the relative contributions of individual drugs, doses, and scheduling. Application of the international prognostic factors may serve to identify those high-risk patients who benefit most from dose- or time-intense approaches and those who do not need intensified treatment.

HIGH-DOSE THERAPY WITH STEM CELL SUPPORT

High-dose chemotherapy followed by stem cell support for progressive or relapsing HL has shown considerable benefit [22–24]. Nevertheless, no advantage of this strategy was seen when compared with conventional chemoradiotherapy as first line treatment.

The European Bone Marrow Transplant Registry conducted a prospective study in poor-risk patients who were randomized to receive high-dose chemotherapy and autografting or an additional four cycles of conventional chemotherapy after achieving CR or partial remission (PR) with four initial cycles of an ABVD-containing chemotherapy. After a median follow-up of 48 months, the 5-year failure-free survival rate was 75% in the high-dose arm and 82% in the conventional arm and the 5-year overall survival rate was 88% in both arms. In conclusion, no benefit from an early intensification for these poor-risk patients was demonstrated [25].

THE ROLE OF CONSOLIDATIVE RADIATION

The role of radiation therapy in advanced HL is controversial [26–29].

The capacity of consolidative radiatio therapy to provide local control in HL is well established. Further, radiotherapy is non–cross-resistant with standard combination chemotherapy. Several authors have reported that approximately 30% of selected patients who relapse after chemotherapy attain durable remission with irradiation [30,31]. The benefits of consolidative radiotherapy must be balanced against the potential for serious late effects, however, particularly second malignancy.

The GHSG conducted the randomized multicenter study HD3 designed to evaluate the role of low-dose (20 Gy) involved-field radiotherapy versus chemotherapy consolidation of complete remission in 288 patients who had advanced HL (see Table 7) [32]. After six cycles of COPP/ABVD, 59% of

Table 8
Results of major randomized trials in adult stage III–IV Hodgkin's lymphoma testing the value of combined modality therapy versus chemotherapy alone

	CR (%)	5-y EFS	5-y survival (%)
SWOG 7808	61	40% CT*	79
		45% CMT*	86
GHSG HD3	59	61% CT	95
		61% CMT	88
GELA H89	50	61% CT*	90
		62% CMT*	83
EORTC 20884	57	48% CT	91
		48% CMT	85

EFS for all patients accrued to trial.
Abbreviations: CMT, combined chemotherapy and irradiation; CT, chemotherapy alone; EFS, event-free survival for all patients accrued to trial; EORTC, European Organization for the Research and Treatment of Cancer; GHSG, German Hodgkin Study Group; GELA, Group d'Etude des Lymphome d'Adulte; SWOG, Southwest Oncology Group.
*Estimated based on CR rate survival for CR pts only.
*Estimated based on published complete response rates.

patients achieved a complete response and 58% of these (34% of the total accrued to study) were randomized to 20 Gy involved-field radiotherapy or two additional cycles of chemotherapy. No significant differences were noted in the study arms either for freedom from progression or overall survival (Table 8). The study had sufficient power to detect a 20% difference after 7 years. Most relapses in both arms of this study were confined to nodal sites of disease. Of interest, the relapse rate was greatest among patients who refused further treatment on either arm of the study.

In the EORTC/GELA #20884 trial, patients who had stage III–IV HL were treated with six to eight cycles of MOPP/ABV [33]. Those who achieved a CR were randomly assigned to receive either involved-field radiotherapy (24 Gy to all initially involved nodal areas, 16–24 Gy to all initially involved extranodal sites) or no further treatment (see Table 7). Among the patients who achieved a CR, 172 received involved-field radiotherapy and 161 received no further treatment. The 250 patients who had PR were all treated with radiotherapy, 30 Gy to PR nodal sites, 24 Gy to CR nodal sites, and 18 to 24 Gy to extranodal sites. The 5-year event-free survival and 5-year overall survival rates were 84% and 91% for patients who had no further treatment and 79% and 85% in the group with CR assigned to involved-field irradiation, $P = .35$ for event-free and $P = .07$ for overall survival (see Table 8). The difference in survival was largely attributed to an increase in secondary leukemia/MDS in the combined modality group (eight cases among 172 patients who had consolidative irradiation, one case among 161 patients after chemotherapy alone).

Among the patients who had PR after chemotherapy, the 5-year event free survival rate was 97% and the 5-year overall survival was 87%, similar to the group of patients who achieved an initial complete response. Interestingly, in this group of 250 patients, there were only two instances of secondary leuke-mia/MDS. These results fail to support the routine use of consolidative irradi-ation in patients who have stage III–IV who achieve a complete response to a full course of conventional irradiation but suggest a beneficial role for those who achieve only a PR.

Another large trial that addressed the specific question of the role of radia-tion therapy for patients who had initially bulky (>5 cm) or residual disease after chemotherapy was the GHSG HD12 study. In this trial, patients were ran-domized to eight cycles of intensified BEACOPP or four cycles intensified BEACOPP plus four cycles of standard BEACOPP followed by either radio-therapy to initial bulky and residual disease or no further treatment. The third interim analysis with 908 patients and a median observation time of more than 24 months showed an FFTF of 90% and an OS of 94% with no significant differences between the treatment arms. In this study, less than 35% of the total cohort of patients received consolidative involved-field radiation [34]. Analysis of the comparison between the radiotherapy (RT) arms and the no RT arms was compromised, because 13% of patients in the no-RT arms of the trial were assigned by a review panel to receive 30 Gy involved-field RT because of either minor response or residual disease greater than 2.5 cm.

The new HD15 trial of the GHSG compares eight cycles of BEACOPP es-calated to six cycles of BEACOPP escalated and eight cycles of BEACOPP-14. In this trial, local RT is given only to PET-positive residual disease.

TOXICITY

A major concern in combined-modality therapy is the potential increase in risk for serious side effects, particularly second malignancy [35]. Difficulties in quantifying the magnitude of risk include the long latency for solid tumors, the important contribution of intensity of drug combinations and cumulative doses, and the radiation variables of field size and dose. These aspects are covered more specifically elsewhere in this issue.

SUMMARY

In 2007, patients who have Hodgkin's lymphoma, even in advanced stages, have a better than 85% chance of being cured of their disease if adequate ther-apy is given at the outset. Adequate therapy today should consider two major principles: risk and response adaptation.

Risk adaptation aims to treat the patient according to the assumed individual risk for treatment failure. The globally used measurement of risk assessment is the IPS. Response adaptation aims to modulate the treatment intensity accord-ing to the observed treatment response, measured by morphologic and functional criteria, such as FDG-PET or CT/PET, during or at the end of treatment.

Most ongoing or planned international studies use these two principles to tailor therapy according to the needs of the individual patient, also accounting for anatomic stage, tumor burden, age, gender, and biologic host factors that affect prognosis. With this approach it might be possible to use less aggressive treatment regimens, such as for the lower risk groups, and limit the use of the more aggressive dose- and time-intensified/dense regimens like BEACOPP-escalated for the higher IPS risk groups. With this individualized approach it might be possible to yield higher cure rates and simultaneously reduce the risk for late complications and mortality.

The remaining question of when, where, and whether at all consolidative radiation should be given may be answered soon by the ongoing international studies using FDG-PET as a predictor of a true complete response after adequate chemotherapy or a PET-positive result that demands further therapy, either radiation or even high-dose chemotherapy, followed by stem cell transplantation.

These issues will only be resolved through well-planned and well-controlled prospective collaborative clinical trials. This compels all oncologists to offer to all patients who have Hodgkin's lymphoma, regardless of clinical stage, the opportunity to participate in clinical trials to improve the outcome for the generations of patients to come.

References

[1] Cheson BD, Pfistner B, Juweid ME, et al. Revised response criteria for malignant lymphoma. J Clin Oncol 2007;25(5):579–86.

[2] Hasenclever D, Diehl V. A prognostic score for advanced Hodgkin's disease. International Prognostic Factors Project on Advanced Hodgkin's Disease [see comments]. N Engl J Med 1998;339(21):1506–14.

[3] Hasenclever D, Loeffler M, Diehl V. Rationale for dose escalation of first line conventional chemotherapy in advanced Hodgkin's disease. German Hodgkin's Lymphoma Study Group. Ann Oncol 1996;7(Suppl 4):95–8.

[4] DeVita VJ, Simon RM, Hubbard SM. Curability of advanced Hodgkin's disease with chemotherapy. Long-term follow-up of MOPP-treated patients at the National Cancer Institute. Ann Intern Med 1980;92:587–95.

[5] Bonadonna G, Zucali R, Monfardini S, et al. Combination chemotherapy of Hodgkin's disease with Adriamycin, bleomycin, vinblastine, and imidazole carboxamide versus MOPP. Cancer 1975;36(1):252–9.

[6] Santoro A, Bonadonna G, Valagussa P. Long-term results of combined chemotherapy-radiotherapy approach in Hodgkin's disease: superiority of ABVD plus radiotherapy versus MOPP plus radiotherapy. J Clin Oncol 1987;5:27–37.

[7] Canellos G, Anderson J, Propert K, et al. Chemotherapy of advanced Hodgkin's disease with MOPP, ABVD, or MOPP alternating with ABVD [see comments]. N Engl J Med 1992;327(21):1478–84.

[8] Viviani S, Bonadonna G, Santoro A, et al. Alternating versus hybrid and ABVD combinations in advanced Hodgkin's disease: ten-year results. J Clin Oncol 1996;14(5):1421–30.

[9] Glick JH, Young ML, Harrington D, et al. MOPP/ABV hybrid chemotherapy for advanced Hodgkin's disease significantly improves failure-free and overall survival: the 8-year results of the intergroup trial. J Clin Oncol 1998;16(1):19–26.

[10] Klimo P, Connors J. MOPP/ABV hybrid program: combination chemotherapy based on early introduction of seven effective drugs for advanced Hodgkin's disease. J Clin Oncol 1985;3(9):1174–82.

[11] Connors J, Klimo P, Adams G, et al. Treatment of advanced Hodgkin's disease with chemo-therapy—comparison of MOPP/ABV hybrid regimen with alternating courses of MOPP and ABVD: a report from the National Cancer Institute of Canada clinical trials group [published erratum appears in J Clin Oncol 1997 Jul; 15(7):2762]. J Clin Oncol 1997;15(4):1638–45.

[12] Duggan D, Petroni G, Johnson J, et al. A randomized comparison of ABVD and MOPP/ABV hybrid for the treatment of advanced Hodgkin's disease: report of an intergroup trial. J Clin Oncol 2003;21:607–14.

[13] Horning SJ, Hoppe RT, Breslin S, et al. Stanford V and radiotherapy for locally extensive and advanced Hodgkin's disease: mature results of a prospective clinical trial. J Clin Oncol 2002;20(3):630–7.

[14] Advani R, Ai WZ, Horning SJ. Management of advanced stage Hodgkin lymphoma. J Natl Compr Canc Netw 2006;4(3):241–7.

[15] Gobbi PG, Levis A, Chisesi T, et al. ABVD versus modified Stanford V versus MOPPEBVCAD with optional and limited radiotherapy in intermediate- and advanced-stage Hodgkin's lymphoma: final results of a multicenter randomized trial by the Intergruppo Italiano Linfomi. J Clin Oncol 2005;23(36):9198–207.

[16] Diehl V, Franklin J, Pfreundschuh M, et al. Standard and increased-dose BEACOPP chemo-therapy compared with COPP-ABVD for advanced Hodgkin's disease. N Engl J Med 2003;348(24):2386–95.

[17] Sieber M, Bredenfeld H, Josting A, et al. 14-day variant of the bleomycin, etoposide, doxo-rubicin, cyclophosphamide, vincristine, procarbazine, and prednisone regimen in advanced-stage Hodgkin's lymphoma: results of a pilot study of the German Hodgkin's Lymphoma Study Group. J Clin Oncol 2003;21(9):1734–9.

[18] Richards M, Waxman J, Man T, et al. EVA treatment for recurrent or unresponsive Hodgkin's disease. Cancer Chemother Pharmacol 1986;18(1):51–3.

[19] Brizel DM, Gockerman JP, Crawford J, et al. A pilot study of etoposide, vinblastine, and doxorubicin plus involved field irradiation in advanced, previously untreated Hodgkin's disease. Cancer 1994;74(1):159–63.

[20] Canellos GP, Gollub J, Neuberg D, et al. Primary systemic treatment of advanced Hodgkin's disease with EVA (etoposide, vinblastine, doxorubicin): 10-year follow-up. Ann Oncol 2003;14(2):268–72.

[21] Friedmann AM, Hudson MM, Weinstein HJ, et al. Treatment of unfavorable childhood Hodgkin's disease with VEPA and low-dose, involved-field radiation. J Clin Oncol 2002;20(14):3088–94.

[22] Chopra R, McMillan A, Linch D, et al. The place of high-dose BEAM therapy and autologous bone marrow transplantation in poor-risk Hodgkin's disease. A single-center eight-year study of 155 patients. Blood 1993;81(5):1137–45.

[23] Horning S, Chao N, Negrin R, et al. High-dose therapy and autologous hematopoi-etic progenitor cell transplantation for recurrent or refractory Hodgkin's disease: anal-ysis of the Stanford University results and prognostic indices. Blood 1997;89(3):801–13.

[24] Reece D, Barnett M, Connors J, et al. Intensive chemotherapy with cyclophosphamide, carmustine, and etoposide followed by autologous bone marrow transplantation for relapsed Hodgkin's disease. J Clin Oncol 1991;9(10):1871–9.

[25] Federico M, Bellei M, Brice P, et al. High-dose therapy and autologous stem-cell transplan-tation versus conventional therapy for patients with advanced Hodgkin's lymphoma responding to front-line therapy. J Clin Oncol 2003;21(12):2320–5.

[26] Hoppe R. Hodgkin's disease–the role of radiation therapy in advanced disease. Ann Oncol 1996;7(Suppl 4):99–103.

[27] Prosnitz L, Wu J, Yahalom J. The case for adjuvant radiation therapy in advanced Hodgkin's disease. Cancer Invest 1996;14(4):361–70.

[28] Loeffler M, Brosteanu O, Hasenclever D, et al. Meta-analysis of chemotherapy versus combined modality treatment trials in Hodgkin's disease. International Database on Hodgkin's Disease Overview Study Group [see comments]. J Clin Oncol 1998;16(3):818–29.

[29] Mauch P. What is the role for adjuvant radiation therapy in advanced Hodgkin's disease? [editorial; comment]. J Clin Oncol 1998;16(3):815–7.

[30] Wirth A, Corry J, Laidlaw C, et al. Salvage radiotherapy for Hodgkin's disease following chemotherapy failure [see comments]. Int J Radiat Oncol Biol Phys 1997;39(3): 599–607.

[31] Pezner R, Lipsett J, Vora N, et al. Radical radiotherapy as salvage treatment for relapse of Hodgkin's disease initially treated by chemotherapy alone: prognostic significance of the disease-free interval. Int J Radiat Oncol Biol Phys 1994;30(4):965–70.

[32] Diehl V, Loeffler M, Pfreundschuh M, et al. Further chemotherapy versus low-dose involved-field radiotherapy as consolidation of complete remission after six cycles of alternating chemotherapy in patients with advance Hodgkin's disease. German Hodgkins' Study Group (GHSG). Ann Oncol 1995;6(9):901–10.

[33] Aleman BM, Raemaekers JM, Tirelli U, et al. Involved-field radiotherapy for advanced Hodgkin's lymphoma. N Engl J Med 2003;348(24):2396–406.

[34] Diehl V. BEACOPP chemotherapy for advanced Hodgkin's disease: results of further analyses of the HD9- and HD12- trials of the German Hodgkin Study Group (GHSG). Blood 2004;104(11):3071.

[35] Mauch P, Ng A, Aleman B, et al. Report from the Rockefeller Foundation Sponsored International Workshop on reducing mortality and improving quality of life in long-term survivors of Hodgkin's disease: July 9–16, 2003, Bellagio, Italy. Eur J Haematol Suppl 2005;(66): 68–76.

Hodgkin's Lymphoma: The Role of Radiation in the Modern Combined Strategies of Treatment

Richard T. Hoppe, MD

Department of Radiation Oncology, Stanford University, 875 Blake Wilbur Drive, Room CC-G224, Stanford CA 94305, USA

At the dawn of the twentieth century, just a few years after Roentgen discovered X-rays, Dr. A. J. Ochsner, a surgeon, referred a young boy who had Hodgkin's disease to William Allen Pusey. Pusey was a professor at the University of Illinois and one of a group of physicians excited by the potential beneficial effects of Roentgen rays. Pusey, a dermatologist, applied them not only to the treatment of cutaneous diseases but also to more deeply situated malignancies. He documented his treatment and observations in the *Journal of the American Medical Association* 2 months later in a paper entitled "Cases of Sarcoma and of Hodgkin's Disease Treated by Exposures to X-rays –a Preliminary Report" [1].

Fortunately for us, in addition to a narrative report of his observations, Pusey published pre- and post-treatment photographs documenting these responses. It is remarkable even today to see the response to treatment of the first person treated with radiation therapy for Hodgkin's disease. The patient was a young boy and his mother reported that he had experienced "eight months of increasing swelling of the glands on the left side of his neck, followed by similar swelling on the right side." Ochsner resected the glands from the right side. When Pusey saw the boy, there was still a massive gland on the left side "as large as a fist. Under x-ray exposures the swelling rapidly subsided and, in two months, the glands were reduced to the size of an almond. At the same time, the general condition of the boy changed from a cachectic, sluggish child to a bright lively one." In another one of his cases included in that same report, Pusey described the effect of the Roentgen ray exposure on the tumor as "almost magical." This was also the first report of combined-modality therapy for the management of Hodgkin's disease, but not in the sense that we currently consider that term.

Later, summarizing his experiences in the 1904 text *The Practical Application of the Roentgen Rays in Therapeutics and Diagnosis*, Pusey concluded that there was no

E-mail address: rhoppe@stanford.edu

0889-8588/07/$ – see front matter
doi:10.1016/j.hoc.2007.06.013
© 2007 Elsevier Inc. All rights reserved.
hemonc.theclinics.com

question as to the beneficial effect of x-rays [2]. He stated that "there can surely be no doubt that cases of Hodgkin's disease should be given the benefit of x-ray exposures as soon as possible after the disease is diagnosed. There seems to be a reasonable hope that, by the use of x-rays, years of usefulness may be added to the lives of these patients."

The second report of the use of x-rays for Hodgkin's disease came from Dr. Nicolas Senn, a professor of surgery at Rush Medical College. In 1903, he reported two cases of pseudoleukemia, a term synonymous with Hodgkin's disease, in the *New York Medical Journal* [3]. One of these patients was a 43-year-old saloonkeeper. Senn wrote that he had "extensive involvement of the glands in both cervical as well as axillary and inguinal regions. He had dullness over the anterior chest and his spleen was considerably enlarged. The patient received 34 treatments and developed the expected dermatitis." Within 1 month of the initiation of treatment, "all of the glands subjected to the x-ray treatment had nearly disappeared."

Impressed by the outcome in the patients he reported in this paper, Senn concluded that "the imminent success attained in these two cases by the use of the x-ray can leave no further doubt of the curative effect of the roentgen therapy in the treatment of Hodgkin's disease. Additional experience will give us more definite information as to the best methods for using the Roentgen ray in the treatment of this disease, with a view of preventing burns and toxic symptoms without reducing its curative effect." This perceptive recognition of the therapeutic ratio has remained a goal in the management of Hodgkin's lymphoma, even today.

But the Roentgen treatment of Hodgkin's disease was to remain a palliative management approach for the next half century. More effective therapy awaited advances in imaging and treatment technology that would allow the more precise identification of disease and more comprehensive radiation treatment with good quality control. The Coolidge tube developed in the 1920s provided a more reliable beam with improved hardness and penetration compared with gas tubes. This made possible the development of orthovoltage x-ray therapy with an energy range of 200 to 250 kV. For many years this was the standard of treatment. Later the 60-Cobalt machine and finally the linear accelerator made curative radiation therapy truly a possibility.

One of the first physicians to extend the concepts of radiation treatment of Hodgkin's disease was Rene Gilbert, a Swiss radiologist. In 1931, Gilbert and Babaiantz published their seminal paper in *Acta Radiologica* describing their method and results of Roentgen therapy for Hodgkin's disease [4]. Gilbert was likely the first to point out the characteristic patterns of the presentation and spread of Hodgkin's disease and to attempt to adapt his treatment techniques to them. He noted that "many times I have seen, in patients recently treated...recurrence developing in the immediate vicinity of a field too narrowly irradiated." He therefore began to advocate irradiation not only to sites of clinical involvement but also to likely sites of microscopic disease adjacent to the involved sites. In the diagrams that Gilbert and Babaiantz published, one can see the primitive forms of the radiation fields that were later adapted as the conventional techniques for treating Hodgkin's disease.

The first person to graphically demonstrate the impact of x-ray treatment on patients with Hodgkin's disease was Dr. C. B. Craft from the University of Minnesota. In 1940, he published a report showing comparative survival for no treatment versus x-ray treatment for patients seen at the University of Minnesota between 1926 and 1939 [5]. He noted that "the difference between the 3 and 5 year survival rates for the treated and untreated groups was highly significant and a testament to the therapeutic value of Roentgen ray therapy. The significant differences should convince even the most dubious of the effectiveness of Roentgen ray therapy in Hodgkin's disease. The patients not only live longer, but their general well-being is tremendously improved in the large majority of cases."

Just as Craft published these observations, secret wartime experiments were being conducted in the United States testing the biologic actions of mustard gas derivatives. Mustard gas had been used in biologic warfare during World War I and was responsible for as many as 400,000 casualties in that conflict. In the early days of World War II, the Chemical Warfare Service of the United States Army began the systematic study of the mustard gases as potential biologic agents. In 1940, Goodman and Gilman at Yale performed pharmacologic studies in rats and noted that the administration of nitrogen mustard was associated with pancytopenia. This finding suggested that the chemical might be useful in treating leukemias and lymphomas. The first patient was treated with nitrogen mustard for lymphosarcoma at the New Haven Hospital in August 1941. Gilman and Philips published the first scientific report regarding this clinical use of nitrogen mustard in the journal *Science* within a year after the close of World War II [6]. They noted that "these studies have revealed a type of action on cells which can be likened to that of no other chemical agent but which resembles in many ways that of x-rays."

Several other reports followed quickly. Goodman and colleagues [7] reported on 27 patients treated for Hodgkin's disease, most of whom "were in advanced or terminal stage of their illness and were considered resistant to Roentgen irradiation." In nearly every case, some benefit was obtained from the treatment. Indeed, the clinical results were sometimes dramatic. Clinical signs and symptoms of disease regressed. They even reported one "patient who did not respond adequately either to radiation or nitrogen mustard therapy alone" in whom "good results were obtained by combining the two agents." Perhaps this was the first actual use of combined chemo–radiation therapy for the treatment of Hodgkin's disease.

Jacobson and colleagues [8] soon reported on 27 patients treated for Hodgkin's disease. They noted that "the rapid resolution of the peripheral, intrathoracic and abdominal lymphadenopathy, the reduction in the size of the spleen and liver and the prompt alleviation of fever and malaise are often striking." One of these cases was a 37-year-old man who had generalized adenopathy, hepatosplenomegaly, and mediastinal involvement. He received six daily treatments between September 7 and September 13, 1943. His response on chest radiograph was dramatic. In addition, his peripheral adenopathy regressed and his systemic symptoms disappeared. The patient was treated intermittently over the next 2.5 years and was still alive without symptoms referable to the disease at the time this report was published.

A paper by Dameshek and colleagues [9], published in the journal *Blood* in 1949, included a detailed analysis of 50 patients who had Hodgkin's disease. For the first time, response to chemotherapy was characterized as partial or complete. The complete response rate for patients who had Hodgkin's disease treated with nitrogen mustard was an incredible 34.3%.

As more experience was accumulated, it was clear that these responses were not durable and, despite repeated therapy, patients inevitably died of their Hodgkin's disease. Lloyd F. Craver was a noted oncologist who practiced at Memorial Hospital in New York. In his reminiscences, entitled "Reflections on Malignant Lymphoma," he noted that "despite all the therapeutic agents that have been added in the past fifteen years, we still need something far better than what we have today. Nitrogen mustard and similar chemical agents have significantly contributed only to palliation. When the future of chemotherapy is spoken of in glowing terms of hope, it must be admitted that it is chiefly in treatment of lymphomas and leukemias that the best results of chemotherapy are seen. And yet in this, the best field, the results are, on the whole, disappointing [10]."

At the same time, the evolution of radiation therapy continued with the work of two preeminent North American radiation oncologists, Dr. Vera Peters from the Princess Margaret Hospital and Dr. Henry S. Kaplan from Stanford. Vera Peters trained with Dr. Gordon Richards at the Ontario Cancer Institute and was a senior radiation oncologist and professor of biophysics and radiology at the University of Toronto. Following up on the early observations of Gordon Richards, Dr. Peters advocated extended-field irradiation in Hodgkin's disease, including prophylactic treatment to sites at high risk for disease. In her analysis of patients treated between 1928 and 1954 with orthovoltage x-rays, she was able to demonstrate an improved outcome with more extended fields and higher doses [11].

Henry Kaplan received an MD from Rush Medical College, trained in radiology at Yale, spent additional time at the National Cancer Institute, and then became Chair of the Department of Radiology at Stanford in 1947. He was the first advocate of high-dose extended-field irradiation for Hodgkin's disease who had the device available to accomplish that treatment—the medical linear accelerator. Based on the observations of Gilbert and Peters, and confirmed by his own analyses of the patterns of disease at presentation and relapse, Kaplan used high-dose extended-field treatment routinely. He then compared his results to patients treated at Stanford by other attending physicians who used a palliative management approach.

At the 1961 meeting of the Radiological Society of North America, Henry Kaplan presented his landmark paper entitled "Radical Radiotherapy of

Regionally Localized Hodgkin's Disease." In this presentation, which was published the following year in the journal *Radiology*, Kaplan showed the dramatic difference in outcome for patients who were treated radically versus those treated palliatively [12]. More than 70% of the patients in the aggressively treated group were free of disease, whereas all of those who were treated with palliative intent had new evidence of disease in less than 4 years.

In the early 1960s at the U.S. National Cancer Institute, following up on early success in the treatment of patients with leukemia using combination chemotherapy, Drs. Tom Frei and Vince DeVita put together a four-drug combination chemotherapy program for the treatment of Hodgkin's disease. Initially this included nitrogen mustard, vincristine, methotrexate, and prednisone. Shortly thereafter, however, a new drug, procarbazine, became available and was substituted for methotrexate, creating the MOPP combination. In their first publication of outcome in 1966, Frei and colleagues [13] reported that patients who had advanced Hodgkin's disease achieved an 86% rate of complete response to MOPP treatment. This finding compared with a rate of only 63% with the combination of vincristine and chlorambucil and 26% with single-agent chemotherapy alone. Later, they reported that 60% of patients who achieved a complete response maintained that response up to 3 years or longer [14], a remarkable achievement for the treatment of advanced Hodgkin's disease.

With these notable advances in chemotherapy and radiation, the stage was set for the introduction of modern combined-modality therapy programs. It is difficult to know who deserves credit for the systematic use of combined modality therapy for Hodgkin's disease, however. In 1954, Lloyd Craver noted that "For the synergistic action of nitrogen mustard and roentgen rays, Karnofsky has been making trials of the injection of a massive dose of nitrogen mustard with the patient on the roentgen-ray therapy table, immediately before the first and rather large dose of roentgen therapy to the local mass of nodes [15]." Karnofsky [16] himself later wrote that he initiated this treatment approach in 1949.

At Stanford, the first use of combined modality therapy was in 1953. In 1957, Frank A. Brown and Henry S. Kaplan wrote in the *Stanford Medical Bulletin* [17] that "in October 1953 a new specific program of treatment for all cases of localized Hodgkin's disease (Stages I and II) was inaugurated by one of us (H.S.K.). This consists of the administration of 0.04 mg/kg nitrogen mustard intravenously, in combination with intensive radiation to the region of involvement. Six cases have thus been treated, and these are briefly summarized here because their freedom from recurrence is sufficiently encouraging to suggest the desirability of a more widespread trial on a controlled basis.

"The rationale for the concurrent use of nitrogen mustard in these localized cases is that it might simultaneously control microscopic, clinically undetectable deposits elsewhere and potentiate the effect of radiation locally. The infrequency with which localized cases of Hodgkin's disease occur even in large institutions suggests the need for cooperative studies in which several therapy centers establish comparative treatment series to which patients are assigned at random after clinical evaluation and staging according to a pre-agreed classification. It is hoped that future studies of this type will clearly reveal whether combined local irradiation and prophylactic chemotherapy, as employed on a trial basis in these six localized cases, significantly increases survival in early Hodgkin's disease [17]." This must have been one of the earliest proposals for prospective randomized clinical trials and cooperative clinical trials groups.

A trial comparing radiation therapy to radiation therapy plus nitrogen mustard was initiated in the United Kingdom in 1959 by Thompson Hancock and Ledlie [18]. Nearly 100 patients were accrued between 1959 and 1965, and the only report of that trial was published as a Preliminary Communication in the journal *Lancet* in 1967. Although they showed an improved survival for combined modality therapy compared with radiation therapy alone, it was not statistically significant.

Credit for the first large-scale implementation of a prospective randomized trial of combined modality therapy for Hodgkin's disease belongs to Dr. Maurice Tubiana. Professor Tubiana organized the European Organization for the Research and Treatment of Cancer (EORTC) cooperative clinical trials group. He chaired the Lymphoma Group and was instrumental in the design of the H1 study for early-stage Hodgkin's disease. The EORTC H1 Study randomized 288 patients who had clinical stage I–II Hodgkin's disease to treatment with radiation therapy alone (a mantle or inverted-Y field) versus radiation followed by 2 years of single-agent vinblastine.

The most recent update of the results of this study show that radiation alone was associated with a risk for treatment failure greater than 60%, whereas patients treated with combined-modality therapy had a risk for treatment failure of only 40%. This difference was statistically significant with a high degree of confidence ($P = .005$). An analysis of survival showed no differences during the first several years of the trial. It was only with a follow-up duration of nearly 25 years that the survival results became significantly different ($P = .04$). In fact, it is unusual for any randomized clinical trial for Hodgkin's disease to demonstrate survival differences, because salvage therapies tend to obliterate any potential differences in survival.

The first clinical trials to explore the potential efficacy of combining high-dose extended-field irradiation with MOPP chemotherapy were the Stanford adjuvant MOPP trials, initiated in 1968. These studies were designed by Drs. Henry Kaplan and Saul Rosenberg [19]. Kaplan had recruited Rosenberg to Stanford in 1961. Saul was a bright young internist who trained in Boston and recently had been a fellow on the Lymphoma Service at Memorial Hospital. He came to Stanford with a joint appointment in the Departments of Radiology and Medicine. Together with Kaplan, in 1962, he first designed trials limited to irradiation, specifically testing the concepts of high-dose extended-field treatment versus more limited palliative therapy. With the introduction of MOPP, however, they quickly developed programs to test combined-modality therapy versus radiation therapy alone for early or intermediate stages of Hodgkin's disease.

One group of the adjuvant MOPP trials tested the value of combined radiation and MOPP chemotherapy for patients who had stage I or II disease. This trial was initiated in 1968 and half the patients were randomized to receive six cycles of adjuvant MOPP therapy following the completion of radiation therapy.

With follow-up extending to nearly 30 years, the difference in freedom from relapse is highly statistically significant. The freedom from relapse at 20 years is 69% for the group treated with radiation alone and 81% for the group treated with combined modality therapy. The survival of both groups of patients was nearly identical, however: 64% and 67% at 20 years. The failure to demonstrate a difference in survival, despite the marked difference in freedom from relapse, was attributable to two factors: (1) patients who relapsed after treatment with irradiation alone had a high likelihood of being salvaged with subsequent MOPP treatment, and (2) patients treated initially with combined modality therapy had a greater risk for treatment-related toxicity, including lethal toxicity, compared with patients treated initially with radiation therapy alone.

The Stanford adjuvant MOPP trials and other similar studies demonstrated that the combination of a full course of radiation therapy and six cycles of chemotherapy could achieve the desired result of an improved freedom from relapse. Long-term survival was similar for either approach, however, and combined-modality therapy was associated with increased complications. This conclusion was mirrored in the meta-analysis published by Specht and colleagues in 1998 [20].

Treatment with combined-modality therapy as it was applied in the 1970s and early 1980s subjected patients to the potential complications and toxicities of all components of therapy. These included infection caused by chemotherapy-related immunosuppression and radiation-related injury of the heart, lungs, thyroid, and so forth. Bone growth and soft tissue abnormalities related to radiation were identified, especially in children. Sterility secondary to MOPP chemotherapy was a virtual certainty for men and affected many women who were older than 30 years. Secondary malignancies included leukemias linked to MOPP and solid tumors related to radiation. Finally, psychosocial problems became apparent in many survivors of Hodgkin's disease treatment. A better approach to combined-modality therapy was needed. An improved therapeutic ratio was required.

Strategies began to be developed to reduce the long-term risks of combined-modality therapy. These included the reduction of radiation fields and doses and the use of safer chemotherapy agents, concepts that provide the current rationale for combined modality therapy in Hodgkin's lymphoma.

FAVORABLE PRESENTATIONS OF STAGE I–II

Favorable presentations of stage I–II include patients who have stage I–II disease who do not have systemic (B) symptoms or large mediastinal adenopathy. In some trials, patients who have an elevated erythrocyte sedimentation rate (ESR) ($\geq$30 or 50), numerous sites of disease ($>$2 or 3), or older age ($>$50) are also excluded and treated according to algorithms for intermediate prognosis. The treatment of choice for favorable prognosis patients is with abbreviated chemotherapy and limited (involved-field) irradiation [21]. Representative trials include the Milan experience of four cycles of Adriamycin, bleomycin, vinblastine, and dacarbazine (ABVD) plus 36 Gy involved-field irradiation (IFRT) [22], the British Trial of vinblastine, Adriamycin, prednisone, etoposide, cyclophosphamide, and bleomycin (VAPEC-B) for 4 weeks, followed by 30 to 40 Gy IFRT [23] and the Stanford trial of 8 weeks of Stanford V chemotherapy followed by 30 Gy IFRT [24].

Important issues that have been addressed in clinical trials include the duration of chemotherapy and the dose of irradiation. In the HD10 trial of the German Hodgkin Study Group (GHSG), patients who had favorable characteristics (normal ESR, no E-lesions, less than three involved regions) were randomized to two versus four cycles of ABVD and 20 versus 30 Gy IFRT [25]. There have been no differences in survival or freedom from treatment failure among the four groups thus far, suggesting that as little as 2 months of chemotherapy and 20 Gy IFRT may be sufficient in this setting.

One of the benefits of the Stanford V program is a reduction in the total doses of chemotherapy. Because chemotherapy complications are largely related to the total doses of individual drugs, this should reduce chemotherapy risks. For example, compared with 4 months of ABVD, the 8-week Stanford V program includes only half the doxorubicin dose (100 versus 200 mg/m^2) and 25% of the bleomycin dose (20 versus 80 mg/m^2). Stanford V includes 120 mg/m^2 of etoposide, but has no dacarbazine. Stanford V does include 12 mg/m^2 of nitrogen mustard, which is the equivalent amount administered in one cycle of MOPP chemotherapy, but has not been associated with sterility or secondary leukemia. Following the completion of Stanford V chemotherapy, patients receive involved-field irradiation to a dose of 30 Gy. This form of management has proved to be effective. The 3-year freedom from progression is 95% and 3-year survival is 97% [26]. The current G5 study uses the same chemotherapy, but reduces the radiation dose to 20 Gy.

Trials that have eliminated radiation therapy entirely have been inconclusive. The National Cancer Institute Canada HD6 trial included arms of ABVD alone, but the comparison arms included subtotal lymphoid irradiation alone for the favorable patients (age>40, lymphocyte predominance or nodular sclerosis histology, ESR>50, and fewer than four involved regions) and 2 months of ABVD followed by subtotal lymphoid irradiation for patients who had any unfavorable characteristics. Although neither radiation therapy–containing arm is currently considered appropriate management, the freedom from progression in the two radiation-containing arms of the trial was superior to that of ABVD alone (93% versus 87%, $P = .006$) [27]. There were no survival differences.

Based on consensus data, the most commonly used treatment for favorable presentations of stage I–IIA Hodgkin's lymphoma is combined-modality therapy with chemotherapy and involved-field irradiation. Selected patients may be considered for treatment with chemotherapy alone if radiation therapy is contraindicated and the increased relapse risk is acceptable. Results of selected studies using combined modality therapy with involved-field irradiation are displayed in Table 1.

UNFAVORABLE PRESENTATIONS OF STAGE I–II

Patients who have unfavorable presentations of stage I–II Hodgkin's lymphoma, usually by virtue of a large mediastinal mass, routinely receive radiation therapy to sites of bulky disease. There is abundant experience with 3 to 6 months of chemotherapy followed by 30 to 40 Gy radiation achieving an excellent outcome. Similar issues remain unanswered as for the favorable presentations (ie, the duration of chemotherapy and the dose of radiation therapy). The GHSG HD11 trial for patients who had intermediate prognosis randomized the chemotherapy to BEACOPP versus ABVD and the radiation therapy dose to 20 versus 30 Gy. No difference in outcome has been reported thus far [28]. This trial was not limited to patients who had large mediastinal adenopathy, however, and included patients who had other adverse factors, including ESR greater than 50, the presence of extranodal disease, and more than two sites of involvement. An analysis has not been performed restricted to patients who had large mediastinal masses. Table 2 [29] displays selected results using combined-modality therapy for patients who had unfavorable presentations of stage I–II Hodgkin's lymphoma.

STAGE III–IV

Several trials have addressed the role of irradiation in the combined-modality management of stage III–IV Hodgkin's lymphoma. The largest and most convincing is the EORTC 20884 trial [30]. In this trial, patients were treated with six to eight cycles of nitrogen mustard, vincristine, procarbazine, prednisone,

Table 1

Representative trials of combined modality therapy (chemotherapy plus involved-field irradiation) for patients who have favorable presentations of stage I–II Hodgkin's lymphoma

Institution/ group	Exclusions	N	Chemotherapy	Radiation dose	FFP (years)	OS (years)
Stanford [26] G4 Trial	B symptoms LMA	87	Stanford V × 8 weeks	30 Gy	96% (8)	98% (8)
Milan [22]		70	ABVD × 4	36 Gy	94% (12)	94% (12)
German Hodgkin Study Group [25] HD 10 Trial	B symptoms Elevated ESR LMA E-lesion >2 sites	1131	ABVD × 2 versus ABVD × 4	20 Gy versus 30 Gy	97% (2)[a]	99% (2)[a]

Abbreviations: FFP, freedom from progression; LMA, large mediastinal adenopathy; N, number; OS, overall survival.

[a] Pooled results from all four arms of the HD10 trial.

Table 2
Representative trials of combined-modality therapy (chemotherapy plus involved-field irradiation) for patients who have unfavorable presentations of stage I–II HD

Institution/ group	Inclusion criteria	N	Chemotherapy	Involved-field radiation dose	FFP (years)	OS (years)
Stanford [26] G2 Trial	LMA	61	Stanford V × 12 weeks	36 Gy	92% (8)	92% (8)
German Hodgkin Study Group [28] HD 11 Trial	B symptoms or elevated ESR or LMA or E-lesion or >3 sites	1363	ABVD × 4 versus BEACOPP × 4	20 Gy versus 30 Gy	90% (2)[a]	97% (2)
EORTC [29] H9U Trial	Age>50 or IIA, ESR>50 or IIB, ESR>30 or >4 sites or LMA	808	ABVD × 4 versus ABVD × 6 versus BEACOPP × 4	30 Gy	91%–94% (4)[b]	93%–96% (4)

Abbreviations: BEACOPP, BEACOPP baseline; FFP, freedom from progression, pooled results from all four arms of the HD11 trial; LMA, large mediastinal adenopathy; N, number; OS, overall survival.
[a] Freedom from treatment failure, pooled results of all arms of the HDII Trial.
[b] Event free survival, range of results from the three arms of the H9U Trial.

Adriamycin, bleomycin, vinblastine (MOPP-ABV) chemotherapy and those who achieved a complete response (CR) were randomized to no further therapy versus 24 Gy IFRT. No differences in freedom from treatment failure (FFTF) or overall survival were identified. In that same trial, however, patients who achieved only a partial response (PR) all received 30 Gy IFRT. The subsequent FFTF and survival for this group closely paralleled the outcome for patients who had achieved a CR, suggesting a value to adding IFRT after a PR has been achieved. Table 3 summarizes the results of the EORTC 20884 trial.

Although the EORTC 20884 trial failed to support the routine use of IFRT after patients achieved a CR to a full course of conventional chemotherapy, there are programs of attenuated chemotherapy in which radiation therapy is retained. The Stanford V program includes only 12 weeks of chemotherapy,

Table 3
Summary results of the EORTC 20884 trial for patients who have stage III–IV Hodgkin's lymphoma

Treatment	Remission status	Consolidation therapy	N	5-year EFS (%)	5-year OS (%)
MOPP-ABV × 6–8	CR	None	161	84	91
MOPP-ABV × 6–8	CR	IFRT 24 Gy	172	79	85
MOPP-ABV × 8	PR	IFRT 30 Gy	250	79	87

Abbreviations: N, Number; CR, Complete response; PR, Partial response; IF RT, Involved field radiation therapy; EFS, Event-free survival; OS, overall survival.
Data from Aleman BMP, Raemakers JMM, Tirelli U, et al. Involved field radiotherapy for advanced Hodgkin's lymphoma. N Engl J Med 2003;348(24):2396–406.

with attenuated total doses of some of the drugs. The schedule of drug administration consists of alternating myelosuppressive and nonmyelosuppressive weeks of therapy. Week one includes doxorubicin, vinblastine, and nitrogen mustard; week two: vincristine and bleomycin; week three: doxorubicin, vinblastine, and etoposide; and week four: vincristine and bleomycin. The cycle is repeated again beginning on week five. Prednisone is continued throughout. It is useful to compare the doses of chemotherapy for 12 weeks of Stanford V versus conventional chemotherapy, for example MOPP-ABV. Compared with 8 months of MOPP-ABV, the 12-week Stanford V program includes only about half the doxorubicin dose (150 versus 280 mg/m^2), one third the bleomycin dose (30 versus 80 mg/m^2), and one third the nitrogen mustard dose (18 versus 48 mg/ m^2). Stanford V includes etoposide, but has no procarbazine. Radiation therapy (36 Gy) is routinely added to initially bulky (>5 cm) sites of disease and to macroscopic splenic involvement [31]. The results of this approach have been excellent [26]. The 12-year freedom from progression is 83% and the 12-year survival is 95%, with only minimal late complications of therapy. The radiation therapy component is essential, however; a study that did not use the same guidelines for radiation therapy resulted in a much worse outcome [32].

RELAPSED DISEASE

There may be a role for radiation therapy in programs of high-dose therapy for salvage after relapse. High-dose chemotherapy and autologous hematopoietic cell rescue is the standard treatment for these patients. Because radiation therapy is so effective in the treatment of Hodgkin's lymphoma, there is compelling reason to incorporate it into these programs, especially if sites of relapse have not been irradiated previously. This has been done in the form of localized irradiation [33] and total lymphoid irradiation [34]. Although randomized trials have not been performed, retrospective data suggest a benefit to the incorporation of radiation therapy in this setting (Table 4) [33].

In this era of combined-modality therapy we have reached the point of near-total conquest of Hodgkin's lymphoma, but challenges remain. There is still

Table 4
Local irradiation as a component of high-dose salvage treatment in relapsed Hodgkin's lymphoma

Patient characteristics	N	3-year FFR (%)		3-year EFS (%)		3-year OS (%)	
		RT	No RT	RT	No RT	RT	No RT
Relapse Stage I–III	62	100	69	85	54	85	67
No prior RT	39	85	57	79	52	93	55

Abbreviations: EFS, event-free survival; FFR, freedom from relapse; N, number; OS, overall survival; RT, radiation therapy.

Data from Poen JC, Hoppe RT, Horning SJ. High-dose therapy and autologous bone marrow transplantation for relapsed/refractory Hodgkin's disease: the impact of involved field radiotherapy on patterns of failure and survival. Int J Radiat Oncol Biol Phys 1996;36(1):3–12.

a small minority of patients who remain resistant to primary therapy and there are others who experience a resistant relapse. In future clinical trials we will likely see more individual adaptation of therapy based on initial prognostic factors and early response criteria, including a response of disease on functional imaging studies, such as 18F-FDG-PET, enabling avoidance of treatment complications for many patients and identifying more accurately those patients who require further intensification of therapy. In addition, newer techniques of irradiation will be explored, such as intensity-modulated radiation therapy [35], involved node irradiation [36], and respiratory gated therapy, all in an attempt to minimize the late effects of therapy.

References

[1] Pusey WE. Cases of sarcoma and of Hodgkin's disease treated by exposures to x-rays— a preliminary report. JAMA 1902;38:166–9.

[2] Pusey WA, Caldwell EW. The practical application of the roentgen rays in therapy and diagnosis. vol. Philadelphia: W.B.Saunders and Co; 1904.

[3] Senn N. Therapeutical value of Roentgen ray in treatment of pseudoleukemia. New York Med J 1903;77:665–8.

[4] Gilbert R, Babaiantz L. Notre methode de roentgentherapie de la lymphogranulomatose (Hodgkin): resultats eloignes. Acta Radiol 1931;12:523–9.

[5] Craft CB. Results with roentgen ray therapy in Hodgkin's disease. Minnesota (MN): University of Minnesota; 1940. p. 401–9.

[6] Gilman A, Philips FS. The biological actions and therapeutic applications of the B-chloroethyl amines and sulfides. Science 1946;103:409–15.

[7] Goodman LS, Wintrobe MM, Dameshek W, et al. Nitrogen mustard therapy. Use of methylbis(beta-chloroethyl) amine hydrochloride for Hodgkin's disease, lymphosarcoma, leukemia and certain allied and miscellaneous disorders. JAMA 1946;132:126–32.

[8] Jacobson LO, Spurr CL, Barron ESG, et al. Studies on the effect of methyl-bis(beta-chloroethyl) amine hydrochloride on neoplastic diseases and allied disorders of the hemopoietic system. JAMA 1946;132:263–71.

[9] Dameshek W, Weisfuse L, Stein T. Nitrogen mustard therapy. Analysis of fifty consecutive cases. Blood 1949;4:338–79.

[10] Craver LF. Reflections on malignant lymphoma; Janeway lecture, 1956. Am J Roentgenol Radium Ther Nucl Med 1956;76(5):849–58.

[11] Peters V. A study of Hodgkin's disease treated radiologically. Am J Roentgenol 1950;63: 299–311.

[12] Kaplan H. The radical radiotherapy of Hodgkin's disease. Radiology 1962;78:553–61.

[13] Frei E, DeVita VT, Moxley JH, et al. Approaches to improving the chemotherapy of Hodgkin's disease. Cancer Res 1966;26(6):1284–9.

[14] Devita VT Jr, Serpick AA, Carbone PP. Combination chemotherapy in the treatment of advanced Hodgkin's disease. Ann Intern Med 1970;73(6):881–95.

[15] Craver LF. Some aspects of the treatment of Hodgkin's disease. James Ewing Memorial Lecture. Cancer 1954;7:927–33.

[16] Karnovsky DA, Miller DG, Phillips RF. Role of chemotherapy in the management of early Hodgkin's disease. Am J Roentgenol 1963;90:968–77.

[17] Brown FA, Kaplan HS. Hodgkin's disease: a revised clinical classification and an approach to the treatment of its localized form. Stanford Med Bull 1957;15:183–90.

[18] Hancock PET, Ledlie EM. Treatment of early Hodgkin's disease. Lancet 1967;1:26–7.

[19] Rosenberg SA, Kaplan HS. The evolution and summary results of the Stanford randomized clinical trials of the management of Hodgkin's disease: 1962–1984. Int J Radiat Oncol Biol Phys 1985;11(1):5–22.

[20] Specht L, Gray RG, Clarke MJ, et al. Influence of more extensive radiotherapy and adjuvant chemotherapy on long-term outcome of early-stage Hodgkin's disease: a meta-analysis of 23 randomized trials involving 3,888 patients. International Hodgkin's Disease Collaborative Group. J Clin Oncol 1998;16(3):830–43.

[21] Hoppe RT, Advani RH, Bierman PJ, et al. Hodgkin disease/lymphoma. Clinical practice guidelines in oncology. J Natl Compr Canc Netw 2006;4:210–30.

[22] Bonadonna G, Bonfante V, Viviani S, et al. ABVD plus subtotal nodal versus involved-field radiotherapy in early-stage Hodgkin's disease: long-term results. J Clin Oncol 2004; 22(14):2835–41.

[23] Moody AM, Pratt J, Hudson GV, et al. British national lymphoma investigation: pilot studies of neoadjuvant chemotherapy in clinical stage Ia and IIa Hodgkin's disease. Clin Oncol (R Coll Radiol) 2001;13(4):262–8.

[24] Horning S, Hoppe R, Breslin S, et al. Very brief (8 week) chemotherapy (CT) and low dose (30 Gy) radiotherapy (RT) for limited stage Hodgkin's disease (HD): preliminary results of the Stanford-Kaiser G4 study of Stanford V + RT, 2000.

[25] Diehl V, Brillant C, Engert A, et al. HD 10: investigating reduction of combined modality treatment intensity in early stage Hodgkin's lymphoma. Interim analysis of a randomized trial of the German Hodgkin Study Group (GHSG). ASCO, 2005.

[26] Horning SJ, Hoppe RT, Advani R, et al. Efficacy and late effects of Stanford V chemotherapy and radiotherapy in untreated Hodgkin's disease: mature data in early and advanced stage patients. Blood 2004;104:92a [abstract: 308].

[27] Meyer RM, Gospodarowicz MK, Connors JM, et al. Randomized comparison of ABVD chemotherapy with a strategy that includes radiation therapy in patients with limited-stage Hodgkin's lymphoma: national cancer institute of Canada clinical trials group and the eastern cooperative oncology group. J Clin Oncol 2005;23(21):4634–42.

[28] Klimm BD, Engert A, Brillant C, et al. Comparison of BEACOPP and ABVD chemotherapy in intermediate stage Hodgkin's lymphoma: results of the fourth interim analysis of the HD 11 trial of GHSG. Paper presented at the Proceedings of the American Society for Clinical Oncology, May 13–17, 2005.

[29] Noordijk EM, Thomas J, Ferme C, et-al. First results of the EORTC-GELA H9 randomized trials: the H9-F trial (comparing 3 radiation dose levels) and H9-U trial (comparing 3 chemotherapy schemes) in patients with favorable or unfavorable early stage Hodgkin's lymphoma. Paper presented at the Proceedings American Society for Clinical Oncology, May 13–17, 2005.

[30] Aleman BMP, Raemakers JMM, Tirelli U, et al. Involved field radiotherapy for advanced Hodgkin's lymphoma. N Engl J Med 2003;348(24):2396–2406.

[31] Horning SJ, Hoppe RT, Breslin S, et al. Stanford V and radiotherapy for locally extensive and advanced Hodgkin's disease: mature results of a prospective clinical trial. J Clin Oncol 2002;20(3):630–7.

[32] Federico M, Levis S, Chisesi T, et al. ABVD versus modified Stanford V versus MOPPEBVCAD with optional and limited radiotherapy in intermediate and advanced stage Hodgkin lymphoma. J Clin Oncol 2005;23:9198–207.

[33] Poen JC, Hoppe RT, Horning SJ. High-dose therapy and autologous bone marrow transplantation for relapsed/refractory Hodgkin's disease: the impact of involved field radiotherapy on patterns of failure and survival. Int J Radiat Oncol Biol Phys 1996;36(1):3–12.

[34] Moskowitz CH, Kewalramani T, Nimer SD, et al. Effectiveness of high dose chemoradiotherapy and autologous stem cell transplantation for patients with biopsy-proven primary refractory Hodgkin's disease. British Journal of Haematology 2004;124(5):645–52.

[35] Loo B, Hoppe RT. Lymphoma: overview. In: Mundt AJ, editor. Intensity modulated radiation therapy. Hamilton, Ontario: BC Decker, Inc; 2005. p. 535–46.

[36] Girinsky T, van der Maazen R, Specht L, et al. Involved-node radiotherapy (INRT) in patients with early Hodgkin lymphoma: concepts and guidelines. Radiother Oncol 2006;79(3): 270–7.

Relapsed and Refractory Hodgkin's Lymphoma: New Avenues?

George P. Canellos, MD

Harvard Medical School, Dana-Farber Cancer Institute, 44 Binney Street,
Boston, MA 02115, USA

R elapse following primary therapy of Hodgkin's lymphoma assumes a similar therapeutic challenge as relapse in any of the lymphomas. It can be categorized into four general groups.

The first is *refractory* disease, representing a failure to achieve a complete or partial remission with initial therapy or outright progression despite therapy. This category represents the most serious example of primary drug or radio resistance and consequently the most difficult to salvage with current cytotoxic agents. Fortunately this represents less than 10% of patients presenting with advanced disease. *Progression* usually refers to increasing evidence of disease after a partial response whose duration may be variable. *Relapse* (or recurrence or disease-free interval) is the reappearance of disease in the original sites or new sites after attainment of an initial complete remission. The timing to relapse has assumed some significance in that the natural history of early relapse from complete remission heralds a more aggressive or refractory pattern of disease than late relapse usually occurring usually after 12 to 18 months of complete remission. *Late relapse* can be further subdivided between asymptomatic, isolated, usually nodal relapse (stage I/II) or disseminated and/or symptomatic relapse. Response criteria for lymphoma have undergone recent revision [1].

It is now a common event to attain long-term progression-free survival in about 90% of patients who present with localized disease usually using combined modality therapy [2–4]. There is also a consideration from several phase II and III trials that chemotherapy alone may achieve a comparable survival but with possibly a slightly higher local recurrence rate that can easily be salvaged. The probability of sparing younger patients the long-term risks of radiation therapy is apparent because about 85% or more of patients treated with chemotherapy alone remain free of disease [5–7]. Patients who have advanced disease are more complicated; 20% to 25% of patients are not likely to achieve a complete remission. Relapse (or treatment failure) varies according to the number of negative prognostic factors determined from the International

E-mail address: george_canellos@dfci.harvard.edu

0889-8588/07/$ – see front matter
doi:10.1016/j.hoc.2007.06.012
© 2007 Elsevier Inc. All rights reserved.
hemonc.theclinics.com

Prognostic Factors Project [8]. Patients who have a prognostic score of 0 to 1 represent about 30% of the total and have a relatively low treatment failure rate of 20%. In the worst prognostic group (four or more factors), which is 19% of the total, the failure rate exceeds 40%. Almost all of that experience refers to patients treated with ABVD (doxorubicin, bleomycin, vinblastine, and dacarbazine) or ABVD/MOPP (nitrogen mustard, vincristine, procarbazine, and prednisone). Prolonged follow-up to 15 to 25 years indicated a somewhat lower event-free survival because of a few late relapses, secondary malignancies, and morbidity related to the toxicity of the therapy [9,10]. Despite these events, the long-term failure-free survival of advanced disease is in the range of 50% to 60% following initial therapy.

The situation is more complicated for patients older than 50 years of age who develop Hodgkin's lymphoma. Although the disease is infrequent in older patients compared with patients younger than 40 years of age, the remission rate, relapse-free survival, and overall survival decrease within each decade after 50 years of age [11,12]. The issue is further complicated by older patients being less likely to tolerate more intensive chemotherapy that often accompanies some salvage treatment programs.

PROGNOSTIC FACTORS AT RELAPSE

The general distribution of relapses from advanced disease treated with initial conventional-dose combination chemotherapy can be assessed from two series of 625 total patients of whom 180 relapsed (28.8%) [13,14]. Of these relapses, induction failures (37.7%) or relapses after less than 12 months (37.7%) were the majority, leaving 24% of the relapses as late (>12 months) failures (Table 1). Using conventional salvage chemotherapy, the Milan group had an 8-year survival overall of 27% with variations from 8% for induction failures to 54% for late relapses.

PRIMARY REFRACTORY DISEASE

Primary refractory (or progressive) disease usually presents with a high order of drug resistance so that no patient in the retrospective analyses by the German Hodgkin's Study Group (GHSG) survived beyond 8 years with salvage conventional-dose chemotherapy only. Using the term primary progressive disease, defined as failure to achieve from complete remission/partial remission (CR/PR) or relapse within 3 months, the response rate to second-line therapy

Table 1
Patterns of relapse in advanced Hodgkin's lymphoma treated with chemotherapy

Series	Total patients	Induction failure	Relapse < 12 months	Relapse > 12 months	Reference
Milan	415	39	48	28	Bonfante et al [13]
Croatia	210	29	20	16	Radman et al [14]
Totals	625	68 (38%)	68 (38%)	44 (24%)	

was 33% but unless high dose with autologous stem cell support was included, all patients died by 5 years. The high-dose salvaged patients had a 43% 5-year survival failure-free in patients who had chemosensitive disease. Chemoresistance and B symptoms at progression were negative prognostic factors. It is clear that all of these patients required high-dose therapy as a component of their salvage treatment. Multivariate analysis would support a 5-year survival of 55% if (1) the Karnofsky score is low at relapse, (2) age is less than 50 years, and (3) a temporary remission to initial therapy is attained. If all three negative factors are present, however, the 5-year survival was 0% in a series of 206 patients [15]. For all patients presenting in relapse, the projected 20-year survival for early relapse was 11% with late relapse accounting for a 22% survival in that study [15]. Similar analysis by the National Cancer Institute (Bethesda) group indicated a poor salvage using conventional-dose chemotherapy [16]. It is noteworthy that ABVD and similar regimens are devoid of classical alkylating agents and inclusion of the latter in salvage therapy may account for the positive results of second-line therapy. Recently more intensive regimens, such as bleomycin, etoposide, adriamycin (doxorubicin), cyclophosphamide, oncovin (vincristine), procarbazine, and prednisone (especially the escalated version), have increased the initial complete response rate and progression-free survival at 5 to 8 years [17]. The increased toxicity is of some concern to clinicians because of the high doses of alkylating agents and etoposide, however. The issue of initial dose intensity might be questioned by the results of a prospective Italian trial that compared ABVD alone to ABVD plus an autologous stem cell transplant as primary therapy. The trial demonstrated no difference in overall survival between the groups [18].

FIRST RELAPSE AFTER ACHIEVING COMPLETE REMISSION WITH CHEMOTHERAPY

The durability of complete remissions achieved by conventional-dose chemotherapy is in the range of 65% to 70% depending on the initial prognostic factors. Some form of salvage therapy, then, is required for 20% to 60% of all patients who have advanced disease treated with initial combination chemotherapy.

When the clinical prognostic factors assessed at the time of relapse are subjected to multivariate analysis several clinical factors are consistent among series. The major negative factors from the Vancouver group (80 patients) include (1) stage IV at initial diagnosis, (2) B symptoms at relapse, and (3) relapse within 12 months. The second time failure-free survival at 5 years with any of these was 17% but 82% if none were present [19]. The GHSG analyzed 422 patients in relapse and created a prognostic score. Independent risk factors were (1) time to relapse, (2) stage at relapse, and (3) anemia. Their overall survival of relapse from radiation only is 89%; early relapse from chemotherapy, 46%; and late relapse from chemotherapy, 71% overall survival [20]. The Hôpital St. Louis analysis (187 patients) focused on two factors: (1) stage III/IV at relapse and (2) relapse after less than 12 months. B symptoms and elevated LDH (lactic dehydrogenase) were also significant but less so than the two major factors [21].

The efficacy of second-line therapy is less in patients who have initial advanced disease treated with chemotherapy than that seen for relapse from radiation therapy alone. Conventional-dose salvage does poorly in some subgroups of relapse. The combined Milan/Croatia series with 625 patients had 5-year survivals of 0%, 8% respectively for induction failures. The overall survival data for early relapse (<12 months) were 28%, 18% and 37%, 54% for late relapse but even in this more favorable group the failure-free survival was only 24%, 44% in those series [13,14]. The Hôpital St. Louis series showed 37% event-free survival at a median of 42 months when conventional-dose salvage therapy was used. It is clear from many series that the use of high-dose therapy can enhance an overall freedom from second failure at 5 years and can range from 46% to 59% [22–25]. Very late relapse is rare but can occur especially in patients who present in clinical stage I/II treated only with radiation therapy. The Princess Margaret Hospital (Toronto) group found that 28% of 731 irradiated patients relapsed overall but only 5% occurred beyond 4 years [26]. This finding confirmed an earlier report from the European Organization for Research and Treatment of Cancer (EORTC) that demonstrated a 3.5% relapse rate beyond 5 years for early Hodgkin's lymphoma treated with radiation therapy [27]. The 10-year survival of very late relapses treated with systemic therapy was 68% in the Toronto series. Late relapse, however defined, thus retains the potential for successful salvage. In one Spanish series, late relapse beyond 2 years occurred in 25 of 223 patients who were in CR at 2 years with 20 of these in continuous remission at a median of 79 months [28]. The EORTC series confirmed a similar long-term salvage of late relapse with 72% 20-year survival.

SALVAGE REGIMENS

Several second- and third-line regimens are actively used to salvage relapsed Hodgkin's lymphoma requiring chemotherapy. Most contain alkylating agents, such as iphosphamide, cisplatinum, and nitrosoureas. More recently gemcitabine has been added to salvage regimens (Table 2). It is difficult to compare the long-term efficacy of the various regimens because a significant fraction of treated patients went on to high-dose therapy with autologous stem cell support. There may be small biologic advantage to relapses following ABVD because the tumor may still be responsive to classic alkylating agents [9]. This situation might explain the relatively high second-line response noted with the various alkylating agent–containing regimens. Four of the more commonly used regimens are ICE (iphosphamide, carboplatin, etoposide) [29], DHAP (dexamethasone, high-dose cytosine arabinoside plus or minus cisplatin) [30], and mini-BEAM (BCNU, etoposide, cytosine arabinoside, melphalan) [31]; when dexamethasone is added at 8 mg every 8 hours from days 1 to 10 then it is referred to as Dexa-BEAM [32]. After gemcitabine was demonstrated to be active as a single agent in relapse, it was incorporated with other agents [33]. The gemcitabine-containing regimens currently in use include: GDC (gemcitabine, dexamethasone, cisplatin) [34]; GEM-P (gemcitabine, cisplatin,

Table 2
Commonly used salvage regimens published since 1995

Drug regimen/reference	Dose, route	Schedule
DEXA-BEAM (German Hodgkin's study group) [32]		
Dexamethasone	8 mg po q 8 h	Days 1–10
Carmustine	60 mg/m^2 IV	Day 2
Etoposide	250 mg/m^2 IV	Days 4–7
Cytarabine	100 mg/m^2 IV q 8 h	Days 4–7
Melphalan	20 mg/m^2 IV	Day 3
Mini-BEAM [31]		
BCNU (carmustine)	60 mg/m^2 IV	Day 1
Etoposide	75 mg/m^2 IV	Days 2–5
Cytarabine	100 mg/m^2 IV q 12 h	Days 2–5
Melphalan	30 mg/m^2 IV	Day 6
Repeated q 4–6 weeks		
ICE [29]		
Ifosfamide	5.0 g/m^2 continuous infusion 24 h (equal dose of Mesna)	Day 2
Carboplatin	AUC 5 IV (max 800 mg)	Day 2
Etoposide	100 mg/m^2 IV	Days 1–3
G-CSF		Days 5–12
Usual 2 cycles with a 2-wk interval		
DHAP [30]		
Dexamethasone	40 mg/m^2 IV	Days 1–4
Cisplatin	100 mg/m^2 IV continuous infusion	Day 1
Cytarabine	2 g/m^2 IV over 3 h q 12 h	Day 2
G-CSF		Days 5–12
GND (CALGB) [36]		
Gemcitabine	1000 mg/m^2	Days 1 and 8
Vinorelbine	15 mg/m^2 IV	Days 1 and 8
Liposomal doxorubicin	10 mg/m^2 IV	Days 1 and 8
Repeated q 21 d		
GDP (Toronto) [34]		
Gemcitabine	1000 mg/m^2 IV over 30 min	Day 1, 8
Dexamethasone	40 mg po	Day 1–4
Cisplatin	75 mg/m^2	Day 1, 8

methylprednisone) [35], and GND (gemcitabine, vinorelbine, liposomal doxo-rubicin) [36]. The response rate to these latter regimens was impressive, in the range of 60% to 65%. The Toronto GDC series, although equivalent to the mini-BEAM experience, demonstrated a relative ease of stem cell collection be-fore transplant and the durability of posttransplant remission was superior. Re-cently a new regimen including iphosphamide, gemcitabine, and vinorelbine

(GEV) was presented by an Italian group showing a 54% CR rate out of 91 patients, including patients who had refractory disease [37].

There are other salvage regimens with more limited experience but which have shown gratifying second-line responses in single publications. They include the usual agents plus some have added or substituted mitoxantrone and idarubicin [38,39].

The most important aspect of second-line therapy is the demonstration of drug responsiveness because outcome of salvage high-dose therapy is predicated on patients achieving a complete or good partial response to second-line regimens. It is noted that the drugs used in high-dose chemotherapy regimens include BCNU, etoposide, cyclophosphamide, high-dose cytosine arabinoside, and melphalan. A good response to conventional-dose salvage regimens usually predicts for a subsequent good response to the high-dose components [40,41].

SALVAGE OF RELAPSE FROM RADIATION THERAPY ALONE

Most patients who relapse following chemotherapy usually do so in prior known sites of disease, whereas irradiated sites tend to have a lower relapse rate and thus recurrences in irradiated patients are more often in the unirradiated marginal areas or disseminated sites. Relapse from primary radiation therapy for stages I/II occurred in 19% to 32% of patients depending on extent and bulk of disease. About 60% occurred in nonirradiated lymph nodes and the remainder in disseminated extranodal sites [26,27]. Initial combined modality therapy for such patients has now eliminated the staging laparotomy and improved the failure rate to 10% to 12%. The relapse rate may be only slightly higher with chemotherapy alone, although the survival is not likely to be compromised [7]. The durability of the remission may also be affected by the extent of radiation if that modality is used alone, but recent studies have confirmed that chemotherapy and limited field radiation is equivalent to the use of the same chemotherapy and more extensive fields of irradiation. In the past, there was a more extensive experience of systemic chemotherapy as a salvage therapy for relapse following radiation therapy alone (Table 3). The impact of combination chemotherapy in primary radiation-only relapses has been favorable, with 10-year survivals in the range of 57% to 89% when ABVD and/or MOPP were used as a salvage regimen [42–46]. It is an unusual circumstance now to

Table 3
Salvage chemotherapy for relapse from primary radiation therapy for stage I–II Hodgkin's lymphoma

Trial site/reference	Patients	Survival
Dana-Farber/Brigham & Women's (Boston) [42]	100	89% (ABVD, 10 y)
Inst. Cura Tumori (Milan) [43]	63	80% (ABVD, 7 y)
Stanford [44]	99	57% (MOPP chemotherapy, 10 y)
Peter McCallum (Australia) [45]	70	71% (MOPP, 10 y)
Royal Marsden (UK) [46]	473	63% (10 y)

see patients in relapse following radiation therapy as their only therapy. The exception to that may be the rare nodular lymphocyte-predominant variant in which local presentations are common, and these can be successfully treated with radiation. Relapses in that disease requiring systemic therapy may occur, however. The optimal cytotoxic regimen is unclear. The unique biology of that variant whereby the tumor cells (lymphocytic/histocytic cells) that are rich with CD20, the B-cell marker on the surface, allow for the anti-CD20 antibody rituximab to have a high order of response in the salvage setting [47,48].

RADIATION THERAPY AS A SALVAGE OF CHEMOTHERAPY RELAPSE

There is an historical experience using radiation therapy as the sole salvage modality for disease recurrent after chemotherapy resulting in a published 23% to 36% failure-free survival at 7 to 10 years. This approach is rarely used in present-day therapy (Table 4) [49–51]. In the two more recent publications a total of 181 patients demonstrated a 75% to 77% complete response rate with excellent infield control (82%). The 5- and 10-year freedom from progression in these selected patients was 28% and 32.8%, respectively [52,53]. Adverse prognostic factors included: (1) male gender, (2) advanced stage at relapse, (3) B symptoms, (4) age greater than 50 years, and (5) less than CR to last chemotherapy. Although these data suggest some value to radiation therapy as a salvage treatment, most patients are likely to receive some form of systemic therapy also. The role of radiation therapy as a component of second-line chemotherapy either before or following high-dose chemotherapy with autologous stem cell infusions is of undefined value, although it is often used [54]. The current approach to salvage therapy should include a consideration of high-dose systemic therapy for almost all groups. The only exception may be a late-occurring isolated asymptomatic relapse. In that setting, the Hôpital St. Louis data suggest that conventional-dose chemotherapy and radiotherapy are likely to be adequate and equivalent to high-dose therapy. There have been only a few trials comparing salvage conventional therapy to that plus high-dose therapy with stem cell support. The European Blood and Marrow Transplant group in a randomized trial showed a superiority in 3-year event-free survival for the transplant arm of 55% versus 34%. There was no statistical overall survival advantage, however [55]. Nonrandomized trials comparing historical series from Stanford demonstrated a 52% 4-year progression-free survival over

Table 4
Radiotherapy alone as a salvage following relapse from chemotherapy

Author/reference	Patients	Median follow-up	Freedom from 2nd relapse
Fox et al (1987) [49]	17	48 mo	24% (5 y)
Brada et al (1992) [50]	25	60 mo	23% (10 y)
Uematsu et al (1993) [51]	14	80 mo	36% (7 y)
Campbell et al (2005) [52]	81	16.8 y	33% (10 y)
Josting et al (2005) [53]	100	52 mo	30% (5 y)

the 19% for conventional-dose therapy [56]. After an analysis of each subgroup of relapses in that series the one that did not show an advantage to high-dose therapy was in those patients who failed late, beyond 12 months.

THE POTENTIAL FOR BIOLOGIC THERAPY

Biologic agents have thus far been used in experimental settings, usually in refractory, heavily treated patients. Currently the sole biologic agent used in the treatment of Hodgkin's lymphoma is the anti-CD20 rituximab antibody, which has been shown to have activity in the CD20-positive nodular lymphocyte-predominant variant whose malignant cells have all of the characteristics of a B-cell neoplasm [47,48].

The major targets that have been the focus of biologic therapeutic investigations are the CD30 antigen, which presents in almost all of the Reed-Sternberg cells of classic Hodgkin's lymphoma, and surface antigens reflective of infection by the Epstein-Barr virus (EBV), which occurs in about 30% of classic Hodgkin's lymphoma.

The CD30 target has been the subject of antibody trials whereby the antibody has been used alone [57,58], linked to another antibody (usually antibody to CD16) [59,60], linked to toxins [61–63], and linked to a radioisotope [64].

There are two recent monoclonal antibodies available for clinical trial: SGN-30 (Seattle Genetics), which is a chimeric antibody, and MDX-060 (Medarex), a fully human IgG antibody. Initial clinical trials with both have shown activity in CD30-positive anaplastic large cell non-Hodgkin's lymphoma and a small number of Hodgkin's lymphoma responses (6 of 12 "stable" with SGN-30 and 3 of 40 responses with MDX-060) [57,58]. The bispecific antibodies (CD30/CD16), with the latter to attract natural killers and cytotoxic T cells, have noted four responses lasting 5 to 9 months out of 16 patients reported in a trial in which IL-2 was co-administered to enhance the response [59]. Another bispecific molecule entailed linking anti-CD30 to a humanized CD64-specific antibody (H22) [60]. In a phase I trial, this immunotherapeutic molecule demonstrated antitumor activity in 4 of 10 patients, one of which was a complete response.

Immunotoxin with the antiCD30 linked to Saporin, a ribosome-inactivating protein, was first reported in 1992 with transient activity in three out of four patients [62]. More recently, anti-CD30 linked to ricin A-chain has been investigated with minimal antitumor activity [61]. Recent investigations have entailed linking the murine CD30 antibody to the radioisotope iodine 131 [64]. Antitumor responses were noted (6 responses out of 22 patients) but responses lasted only about 5 months. Development has been slow despite a variety of isotopes and toxins available for linkage.

To the lesser extent, the receptor for IL-2, CD25, has been a target for biologic therapy with a fusion molecule of IL-2 toxin (diphtheria toxin) with limited clinical trials [65].

The presence of specific EBV-related surface antigens, LMP1 and LMP2A, has permitted the generation of autologous LMP2-specific cytotoxic T lymphocytes ex vivo to be used in relapsed EBV-positive lymphoma. Preliminary experience indicated safety and some antitumor activity, but the process does require ex vivo generation of LMP2 cytotoxic lymphocytes using genetically modified lymphoblastoid cell lines to prime the autologous lymphocytes [66]. The technique has been investigated as a treatment of EBV-related lymphoproliferative disorders in solid organ transplant patients [67]. The EBV-related LMP1 epitope has also been incorporated into a pox virus vaccine with the intent to develop active vaccination against EBV-related malignancies [68]. Other cellular immunotherapeutics include the reinfusion of donor leukocytes to patients following allogeneic transplantation but with progressive disease. Responses were noted in four of nine patients lasting a median of 7 months, but almost all developed graft-versus-host disease [69]. Biologic therapeutics is still investigational, but the rapid pace of new biologic insights into the biology of the malignant Hodgkin's lymphoma cell should reveal new targets for the development of specific agents [70].

References

[1] Cheson BD, Pfistner B, Juweid M, et al. Revised response criteria for malignant lymphoma. J Clin Oncol 2007;25:579–86.

[2] Bonadonna G, Bonfante V, Viviani S, et al. ABVD plus subtotal nodal versus involved-field radiotherapy in early-stage Hodgkin's disease: long-term results. J Clin Oncol 2004;22: 2835–41.

[3] Engert A, Schiller P, Josting A, et al. Involved-field radiotherapy is equally effective and less toxic compared with extended-field radiotherapy after four cycles of chemotherapy in patients with early-stage unfavorable Hodgkin's lymphoma: results of the HD8 trial of the German Hodgkin's Lymphoma study group. J Clin Oncol 2003;21:3601–8.

[4] Brusamolino E, Baio A, Orlandi E, et al. Long-term events in adult patients with clinical stage IA-IIA nonbulky Hodgkin's lymphoma treated with four cycles of doxorubicin, bleomycin, vinblastine, and dacarbazine and adjuvant radiotherapy: a single-institution 15-year follow-up. Clin Cancer Res 2006;12:6487–93.

[5] Straus DJ, Portlock CS, Qin J, et al. Results of a prospective randomized clinical trial of doxorubicin, bleomycin, vinblastine, and dacarbazine (ABVD) followed by radiation therapy (T) versus ABVD alone for stages I, II and IIIA nonbulky Hodgkin disease. Blood 2004;104: 3483–9.

[6] Dominguez AR, Marquez A, Guma J, et al. Treatment of stage I and II Hodgkin's lymphoma with ABVD chemotherapy: results after 7 years of a prospective study. Ann Oncol 2004;15: 1798–804.

[7] Meyer RM, Gospodarowicz MK, Connors JM, et al. Randomized comparison of ABVD chemotherapy with a strategy that includes radiation therapy in patients with limited-stage Hodgkin's lymphoma: National Cancer Institute of Canada clinical trials group and the Eastern Cooperative Oncology Group. J Clin Oncol 2005;23:4634–42.

[8] Hasenclever D, Diehl V. A prognostic score for advanced Hodgkin's disease. N Engl J Med 1998;339:1506–14.

[9] Canellos GP, Anderson JR, Propert KJ, et al. Chemotherapy of advanced Hodgkin's disease with MOPP, ABVD or MOPP alternating with ABVD. N Engl J Med 1992;327: 1478–84.

[10] Canellos GP, Niedzwiecki D. Long-term follow-up of Hodgkin's disease trial. N Engl J Med 2002;3346:1417–8.

[11] Stark GL, Wood KM, Jack F, et al. Hodgkin's disease in the elderly: a population-based study. Br J Haematol 2002;119:432–40.

[12] Engert A, Ballova V, Haverkamp H, et al. Hodgkin's lymphoma in elderly patients: a compre-hensive retrospective analysis from the German Hodgkin's study group. J Clin Oncol 2005;23:5052–60.

[13] Bonfante V, Santoro A, Viviani S, et al. Outcome of patients with Hodgkin's disease failing after primary MOPP-ABVD. J Clin Oncol 1997;15:528–34.

[14] Radman I, Basic N, Labar B, et al. Long-term results of conventional-dose salvage chemother-apy in patients with refractory and relapsed Hodgkin's disease (Croatian experience). Ann Oncol 2002;13:1650–5.

[15] Josting A, Rueffer U, Franklin J, et al. Prognostic factors and treatment outcome in primary progressive Hodgkin lymphoma: a report from the German Hodgkin Lymphoma study group. Blood 2000;96:1280–6.

[16] Longo DL, Duffey PL, Young RC, et al. Conventional-dose salvage combination chemother-apy in patients relapsing with Hodgkin's disease after combination chemotherapy: the low probability for cure. J Clin Oncol 1992;10:210–8.

[17] Diehl V, Franklin J, Pfreundschuh M, et al. Standard and increased-dose BEACOPP chemo-therapy compared with COPP-ABVD for advanced Hodgkin's disease. N Engl J Med 2003;348:2386–95.

[18] Federico M, Bellei M, Brice P, et al. High-dose therapy and autologous stem-cell transplan-tation versus conventional therapy for patients with advanced Hodgkin's lymphoma re-sponding to front-line therapy. J Clin Oncol 2003;21:2320–5.

[19] Lohri A, Barnett M, Fairey RN, et al. Outcome of treatment of first relapse of Hodgkin's dis-ease after primary chemotherapy: identification of risk factors from the British Columbia ex-perience 1970 to 1988. Blood 1991;77:2292–8.

[20] Josting A, Franklin J, May M, et al. New prognostic score based on treatment outcome of patients with relapsed Hodgkin's lymphoma registered in the database of the German Hodgkin's Lymphoma study group. J Clin Oncol 2001;20:221–30.

[21] Brice P, Bastion Y, Divine M, et al. Analysis of prognostic factors after the first relapse of Hodgkin's disease in 187 patients. Cancer 1996;78:1293–9.

[22] Moskowitz CH, Kewalramani T, Nimer SD, et al. Effectiveness of high dose chemoradiother-apy and autologous stem cell transplantation for patients with biopsy-proven primary refrac-tory Hodgkin's disease. Br J Haematol 2004;124:645–52.

[23] Josting A, Rudolph C, Mapara M, et al. Cologne high-dose sequential chemotherapy in relapsed and refractory Hodgkin lymphoma: results of a large multicenter study of the German Hodgkin Lymphoma Study Group (GHSG). Ann Oncol 2005;16:116–23.

[24] Ferme C, Mounier N, Divine M, et al. Intensive salvage therapy with high-dose chemother-apy for patients with advanced Hodgkin's disease in relapse or failure after initial chemo-therapy: results of the Groupe d'Etudes des Lymphomes de l'Adulte H89 trial. J Clin Oncol 2002;20:467–75.

[25] Lazarus HM, Loberiza F, Zhang M-J, et al. Autotransplants for Hodgkin's disease in first re-lapse or second remission: a report from the autologous blood and marrow transplant reg-istry (ABMTR). Bone Marrow Transplant 2001;27:387–96.

[26] Brierley JD, Rathmel AJ, Gospodarowicz MK, et al. Late relapse after treatment for clinical stage I and II Hodgkin's disease. Cancer 1997;79:1422–7.

[27] Bodis S, Henry-Amar M, Bosq J, et al. Late relapse in early-stage Hodgkin's disease patients enrolled on European organization for research and treatment of cancer protocols. J Clin Oncol 1993;11:225–32.

[28] Garcia-Carbonero R, Paz-Ares L, Arcediano A, et al. Favorable prognosis after late relapse of Hodgkin's disease. Cancer 1998;83:560–5.

[29] Moskowitz CH, Nimer SD, Zelenetz AD, et al. A 2-step comprehensive high-dose chemoradiotherapy second-line program for relapsed and refractory Hodgkin disease: analysis by intent to treat and development of prognostic model. Blood 2001;97:616–23.

[30] Josting A, Rudolph C, Reiser M, et al. Time-intensified dexamethasone/cisplatin/cytara-bine: an effective salvage therapy with low toxicity in patients with relapsed and refractory Hodgkin's disease. Ann Oncol 2002;13:1628–35.

[31] Martin A, Fernandez-Jimenez MC, Caballero MD, et al. Long-term follow-up in patients treated with Mini-BEAM as salvage therapy for relapsed or refractory Hodgkin's disease. Br J Haematol 2001;113:161–71.

[32] Pfreundschuh MG, Rueffer U, Lathan B, et al. Dexa-BEAM in patients with Hodgkin's disease refractory to multidrug chemotherapy regimens: a trial of the German Hodgkin's Disease study group. J Clin Oncol 1994;12:580–6.

[33] Santoro A, Bredenfeld H, Devizzi L, et al. Gemcitabine in the treatment of refractory Hodg-kin's disease: results of a multicenter phase II study. J Clin Oncol 2000;18:2615–9.

[34] Kuruvilla J, Nagy T, Pintilie M, et al. Similar response rates and superior early progression-free survival with gemcitabine, dexamethasone, and cisplatin salvage therapy compared with carmustine, etoposide, cytarabine, and melphalan salvage therapy prior to autologous stem cell transplantation for recurrent or refractory Hodgkin lymphoma. Cancer 2006;106: 353–60.

[35] Chau I, Harries M, Cunningham D, et al. Gemcitabine, cisplatin and methylprednisolone chemotherapy (GEM-P) is an effective regimen in patients with poor prognostic primary pro-gressive or multiply relapsed Hodgkin's and non-Hodgkin's lymphoma. Br J Haematol 2003;120:970–7.

[36] Bartlett N, Niedzwiecki D, Johnson J, et al. A phase I/II study of gemcitabine, vinorelbine, and liposomal doxorubicin for relapsed Hodgkin's disease. Proc Am Soc Clin Oncol 2003;22:141 [abstract #2275].

[37] Santoro A, Magagnali M, Spina M, et al. Ifosfamide, gemcitabine, and vinorelbine: a new regimen for refractory and relapsed Hodgkin's lymphoma. Haematologica 2007;92: 35–41.

[38] Alexandrescu DT, Karri S, Wiernik PH, et al. Mitoxantrone, vinblastine and CCNU: long-term follow-up of patients treated for advanced and poor-prognosis Hodgkin's disease. Leuk Lymphoma 2006;47:641–56.

[39] Oyan B, Koc Y, Ozdemir E, et al. Ifosfamide, idarubicin, and etoposide in relapsed/refrac-tory Hodgkin disease or non-Hodgkin lymphoma: a salvage regimen with high response rates before autologous stem cell transplantation. Biol Blood Marrow Transplant 2005;11:688–97.

[40] Majhail NS, Weisdorf DJ, Defor TE, et al. Long-term results of autologous stem cell transplan-tation for primary refractory or relapsed Hodgkin's lymphoma. Biol Blood Marrow Trans-plant 2006;12:1065–72.

[41] Sureda A, Constans M, Irionda A, et al. Prognostic factors affecting long-term outcome after stem cell transplantation in Hodgkin's lymphoma autografted after a first relapse. Ann Oncol 2005;16:625–33.

[42] Ng AK, Li S, Neuberg D, et al. Comparison of MOPP versus ABVD as salvage therapy in patients who relapse after radiation therapy alone for Hodgkin's disease. Ann Oncol 2004;15:270–5.

[43] Santoro A, Viviana S, Villarreal CJR. Salvage chemotherapy in Hodgkin's disease irradia-tion failures: superiority of doxorubicin-containing regimens over MOPP. Cancer Treat Rep 1986;15(2):528–34.

[44] Roach M, Brophy N, Cox R, et al. Prognostic factors for patients relapsing after radiotherapy for early-stage Hodgkin's disease. J Clin Oncol 1990;8:623–9.

[45] Olver IN, Wolf MM, Cruickshank D, et al. Nitrogen mustard, vincristine, procarbazine, and prednisolone for relapse after radiation in Hodgkin's disease. An analysis of long-term fol-low-up. Cancer 1988;62:233–9.

[46] Horwich A, Spect L, Ashley S. Survival analysis of patients with clinical stages I or II Hodg-kin's disease who have relapsed after initial treatment with radiotherapy alone. Eur J Cancer 1997;33:848–53.

[47] Ekstrand BC, Lucas JB, Horwitz SM, et al. Rituximab in lymphocyte-predominant Hodgkin disease: results of a phase 2 trial. Blood 2003;101:4285–9.

[48] Rehwald U, Schulz H, Reiser M, et al. Treatment of relapsed CD20+ Hodgkin lymphoma with the monoclonal antibody rituximab is effective and well tolerated: results of a phase 2 trial of the German Hodgkin Lymphoma study group. Blood 2003;101: 420–4.

[49] Fox KA, Lippman SM, Cassady JR, et al. Radiation therapy salvage of Hodgkin's disease following chemotherapy failure. J Clin Oncol 1987;5:38–45.

[50] Brada M, Eeles R, Ashley S, et al. Salvage radiotherapy in recurrent Hodgkin's disease. Ann Oncol 1992;3:131–5.

[51] Uematsu M, Tarbell NJ, Silver B, et al. Wide-field radiation therapy with or without chemotherapy for patients with Hodgkin disease in relapse after initial combination chemotherapy. Cancer 1993;72:207–12.

[52] Campbell B, Wirth A, Milner A, et al. Long-term follow-up of salvage radiotherapy in Hodgkin's lymphoma after chemotherapy failure. Int J Radiat Oncol Biol Phys 2005;63: 1538–45.

[53] Josting A, Nogova L, Franklin J, et al. Salvage radiotherapy in patients with relapsed and refractory Hodgkin's lymphoma: a retrospective analysis from the German Hodgkin Lymphoma study group. J Clin Oncol 2005;23:1522–9.

[54] Wendland MMM, Asch JD, Pulsipher MA, et al. The impact of involved field radiation therapy for patients receiving high-dose chemotherapy followed by hematopoietic progenitor cell transplant for the treatment of relapsed or refractory Hodgkin disease. Am J Clin Oncol 2006;29:189–95.

[55] Schmitz N, Pfistner B, Sextro M, et al. Aggressive conventional chemotherapy compared with high-dose chemotherapy with autologous haemopoietic stem-cell transplantation for relapsed chemosensitive Hodgkin's disease: a randomized trial. Lancet 2002;359: 2065–71.

[56] Yuen A, Rosenberg SA, Hoppe RT, et al. Comparison between conventional salvage therapy and high-dose therapy with autografting for recurrent or refractory Hodgkin's disease. Blood 1997;89:814–22.

[57] Leonard J, Rosenblatt JD, Bartlett NL, et al. Phase II study of SGN-30 (anti-CD30 monoclonal antibody patients with refractory or recurrent Hodgkin's disease. Blood 2004;104:721a [abstract #2635].

[58] Ansell SM, Byrd JC, Horwitz SM, et al. Phase I/II open-label dose-escalating study of MDX-060 administered weekly for 4 weeks in subjects with refractory/relapsed CD30 positive lymphoma. Blood 2004;104:721a [abstract #2636].

[59] Hartmann F, Renner C, Jung W, et al. Anti-CD16/CD30 bispecific antibody treatment for Hodgkin's disease: role of infusion schedule and costimulation with cytokines. Clin Cancer Res 1973;7:1873–81.

[60] Borchmann P, Schnell R, Fuss I, et al. Phase I trial of the novel bispecific molecule H22xKi-4 in patients with refractory Hodgkin lymphoma. Blood 2002;100:3101–7.

[61] Schnell R, Staak O, Borchmann P, et al. A phase I study with an anti-CD30 ricin A-chain immunotoxin (Ki-4.dgA) in patients with refractory CD30+ Hodgkin's and non-Hodgkin's lymphoma. Clin Can Res 2002;8:1779–86.

[62] Falini B, Bolognesi A, Flenghi L, et al. Response of refractory Hodgkin's disease to monoclonal anti-CD30 immunotoxin. Lancet 1992;339:1195–6.

[63] Engert A, Diehl V, Schnell R, et al. A phase-I study of an anti-CD25 ricin A-chain immunotoxin (RFT5-SMPT-dgA) in patients with refractory Hodgkin's lymphomas. Blood 1997;89: 403–10.

[64] Schnell R, Dietlein M, Staak JO, et al. Treatment of refractory Hodgkin's lymphoma patients with an iodine-131-labeled murine anti-CD30 monoclonal antibody. J Clin Oncol 2005;23: 4669–78.

[65] Tepler I, Schwartz G, Parker K, et al. Phase I trial of an interleukin-2 fusion toxin (DAB486IL-2) in hematologic malignancies: complete response in a patient with Hodgkin's disease refractory to chemotherapy. Cancer 1994;73:1276–85.

[66] Su Z, Peluso MV, Raffegerst SH, et al. The generation of LMP2a-specific cytotoxic T lymphocytes for the treatment of patients with Epstein-Barr virus-positive Hodgkin disease. Eur J Immunol 2001;31:947–58.

[67] Comoli P, Labirio M, Basso S, et al. Infusion of autologous Epstein-Barr virus (EBV)-specific cytotoxic T cells for prevention of EBV-related lymphoproliferative disorder in solid organ transplant recipients with evidence of active virus replication. Blood 2002;99:2592–8.

[68] Duralswamy J, Sherritt M, Thomson S, et al. Therapeutic LMP1 polyepitope vaccine for EBV-associated Hodgkin disease and nasopharyngeal carcinoma. Blood 2003;101:3150–6.

[69] Anderlini P, Acholonu SA, Okoroji G-J, et al. Immunotherapy with donor leukocyte infusions (DLIS) in relapsed Hodgkin's disease (HD) following allogeneic stem cell transplantation (ALLO-SCT): CD3+ cell dose, GVHD and disease response. Blood 2004;104:460a [abstract #1654].

[70] Re D, Thomas RK, Behringer K, et al. From Hodgkin disease to Hodgkin lymphoma: biologic insights and therapeutic potential. Blood 2005;105:4553–60.

Autologous and Allogeneic Stem Cell Transplantation in Hodgkin's Lymphoma

Anna Sureda, MD, PhD

Department of Hematology, Clinical Hematology Division, Hospital de la Santa Creu i Sant Pau, Antoni Maria i Claret, 167, 08025 Barcelona, Spain

Newly diagnosed patients who have advanced-stage Hodgkin's lymphoma (HL) have an excellent prognosis because most of them can be cured with initial treatment [1]. In contrast, the prognosis for patients relapsing after first-line therapy with either combination chemotherapy or chemotherapy followed by radiotherapy remains poor in many cases. In most of these cases, high-dose chemotherapy and autologous stem cell transplantation (ASCT) is nowadays considered to be the treatment of choice.

AUTOLOGOUS STEM CELL TRANSPLANTATION IN REFRACTORY/RELAPSED HODGKIN'S LYMPHOMA

Prognostic Factors at Relapse for Autologous Stem Cell Transplant Recipients

Several attempts have been made to construct prognostic indexes at relapse with the objective of identifying subgroups of patients with a poor outcome with a conventional ASCT. Inconsistent findings among studies are attributable to small patient numbers, inclusion of patients with primary refractory disease (PRD), and, in some series, lack of multivariate analysis.

In a series of 128 patients who had relapsed HL homogeneously treated with the cyclophosphamide, carmustine, etoposide (CBV) protocol, Bierman and colleagues [2] found that a poor performance status, failure of two or more chemotherapy protocols, and the presence of mediastinal disease predicted a poor outcome after ASCT, with a 4-year failure-free survival of only 10% in those patients failing two or more protocols. Reece and colleagues [3] reported an analysis of 58 patients treated with ASCT in a single institution. Four prognostic groups were identified, according to the presence of the following parameters at relapse: B symptoms, extranodal disease, and a short first complete remission (CR). Patients with no risk factors had a 3-year progression-free survival (PFS) of 100%, compared with 81% for patients with one risk factor,

E-mail address: asureda@santpau.es

0889-8588/07/$ – see front matter
doi:10.1016/j.hoc.2007.07.008

© 2007 Elsevier Inc. All rights reserved.
hemonc.theclinics.com

40% for those with two risk factors, and finally, 0% for patients with three risk factors.

In patients autografted with the CBV protocol or the combination of total body irradiation (TBI)-cyclophosphamide and etoposide, the group of City of Hope showed that more than two prior chemotherapy protocols, prior radiotherapy, and extranodal disease at ASCT predicted a poor outcome after the procedure [4]. Similarly, in a group that included 119 relapsed or refractory HL patients autografted with the same regimens, the combination of B symptoms at relapse, BM or pulmonary involvement at ASCT, and the presence of lymph nodes greater than or equal to 2 cm were able to separate different prognostic groups, with a 4-year event-free survival (EFS) of 85% for patients with no adverse prognostic factors, compared with 41% for patients with one bad prognostic factor [5].

The French cooperative group GELA analyzed the prognostic factors at relapse after a first CR in a group of 280 patients undergoing an ASCT [6]. They developed a two-factor model incorporating a short first CR and the presence of extranodal disease at relapse as adverse prognostic factors. With this model, patients with zero, one, or two risk factors presented PFS rates of 93%, 59%, and 43%, respectively. The Memorial Sloan-Kettering Cancer Center investigators [7] have developed a prognostic model of risk factors at relapse (B symptoms, extranodal disease, and CR duration of less than 1 year) in a group of 65 patients (22 PRD and 43 relapsed) treated with two bi-weekly cycles of ifosfamide, carboplatin, and etoposide. The presence of zero to one risk factor was associated with an EFS rate of 83%, whereas it decreased to 10% in patients presenting with the three risk factors. This prognostic model has been used to develop tailored therapeutic strategies [8]. The Spanish GEL/TAMO co-operative group, in a series of 357 patients who had relapsed HL after a first CR, found that advanced stage at diagnosis, radiotherapy before ASCT, a short first CR, and detectable disease at ASCT adversely influenced time to treatment failure (TTF); year of transplantation (before 1996), bulky disease at diagnosis, a short first CR, detectable disease at ASCT and one or more extranodal areas involved at ASCT were adverse factors for overall survival (OS) [9].

Finally, in the largest series to date, Josting and colleagues [10], from the German Hodgkin Lymphoma Study Group (GHSG), developed a prognostic score for relapsed HL, based on outcomes of 471 patients who failed primary therapy. In multivariate analysis, independent risk factors were time to relapse (12 months versus >12 months), clinical stage at relapse (stage III or IV), and anemia at relapse (males <12 g/dL; females <10.5 g/dL). Five-year freedom from second failure rates for patients failing primary chemotherapy or combined modality therapy were approximately 45%, 32%, and 18% for patients with prognostic scores of 0 to 1, 2, and 3, respectively. Only 8% of patients had all three poor prognostic factors, with 70% having a score of 0 to 1. This prognostic score worked well in patients relapsing after chemotherapy or radiotherapy and therefore was considered to be broadly applicable in guiding clinical decision making.

Autologous Stem Cell Transplantation for Relapsed Hodgkin's Lymphoma

The use of ASCT is now considered the standard of care for relapsed HL patients [11]. In several phase II studies, ASCT has been shown to produce between 30% and 65% long-term disease-free survival in selected patients with refractory and relapsed HL [2–4,12–16]. Two randomized trials showed significant benefit in freedom from treatment failure (FFTF) for ASCT over conventional chemotherapy for relapsed disease [17,18]. These trials have resulted in the recommendation of ASCT at the time of first relapse for even the most favorable patients, although salvage radiotherapy can offer an effective treatment for selected subsets of patients who have relapsed or refractory HL [19]. The lack of a survival benefit in these randomized trials has been attributed to patients in the nontransplant arm undergoing transplantation at the time of second relapse.

Randomized trials

The first randomized trial of transplantation for relapsed disease was a small trial from the British National Lymphoma Investigation, comparing ASCT with BCNU, etoposide, ara-C, and melphalan (BEAM) as a preparative regimen to mini-BEAM without autologous transplantation [17] in patients who had active HL, for whom conventional therapy had failed. Twenty patients were assigned treatment with BEAM plus ASCT, and 20, mini-BEAM. All had been followed up for at least 12 months (median 34 months). Five BEAM recipients died (two from causes related to ASCT and three from disease progression), compared with nine mini-BEAM recipients (all disease progression). The difference was not significant ($P = .318$). However, both 3-year EFS and PFS showed significant differences in favor of BEAM plus ASCT ($P = .025$ and $P = .005$, respectively). The study showed no differences in OS. This trial was prematurely closed because recruitment became increasingly difficult as patients refused randomization and requested an ASCT.

In the second randomized trial performed by investigators of the GHSG and the Lymphoma Working Party (WP) of the European Group for Blood and Marrow Transplantation (EBMT), 161 patients between 16 and 60 years of age with relapsed HL were randomly assigned two cycles of Dexa-BEAM (dexamethasone and carmustine, etoposide, cytarabine, and melphalan) and either two further courses of Dexa-BEAM or high-dose BEAM and transplantation of hemopoietic stem cells [18]. Only patients who had chemosensitive disease (CR or partial remission [PR]) after two courses of Dexa-BEAM proceeded to further treatment. Of the 117 patients who had chemosensitive relapse, 3-year FFTF was significantly improved for patients undergoing ASCT compared with four cycles of Dexa-BEAM (55% versus 34%, $P = .019$). With a median follow-up of 39 months (range, 3–78), the 3-year FFTF was significantly better for patients treated with BEAM, regardless of whether first relapse had occurred early (<12 months) (41% versus 12%, $P = .007$) or late (>12 months) (75% versus 44%, $P = .02$) (Figs. 1 and 2). No significant

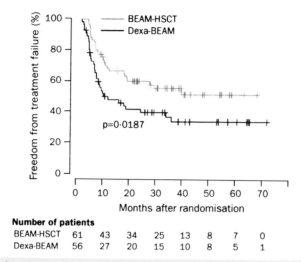

Fig. 1. FFTF for patients who have relapsed chemosensitive HL. HSCT, hematopoietic stem cell transplantation.

improvement of ASCT over conventional salvage chemotherapy in terms of FFTF could be observed in the small subgroup of patients treated for multiple-relapsed disease (n = 24). No subgroup of patients showed a statistically significant difference in OS (Fig. 3). After a median follow-up of 7 years, results continue to show an advantage for high-dose therapy (49% versus 32%, $P = .02$) but still no difference in 7-year OS rates. The absence of differences in OS might be partly because about one third of the patients receiving conventional salvage chemotherapy received an ASCT after further relapse. As in the first reported analysis, patients with multiple relapses before trial entry showed no differences in 7-year FFTF (32% for Dexa-BEAM versus 27% for BEAM-hematopoietic stem cell transplantation). No excess rate of myelodysplastic syndromes/secondary acute myelogenous leukemia was reported in the high-dose arm [19].

To improve the results of ASCT in relapsed or refractory HL patients, the GHSG has used a sequential high-dose chemotherapy before the intensive procedure [20]. Treatment started with two cycles of cisplatin, high-dose cytarabine, and dexamethasone to reduce tumor burden. Patients achieving a CR or PR subsequently received a high-dose chemotherapy program with cyclophosphamide (4 g/m^2 IV), methotrexate (8 g/m^2 IV), vincristine (1.4 mg/m^2 IV) and etoposide (2 g/m^2 IV). Patients were then autografted using the BEAM protocol. Response rate after the final evaluation was 80% (72% CR, 8% PR). With a median follow-up of 40 months (range, 3–84), FFTF and OS for patients with early relapse were 62% and 78%, respectively, and for patients with late relapse, 63% and 79%, respectively. This promising approach is being investigated in a phase III prospective randomized trial between the GHSG and the Lymphoma WP of the EBMT (*HDR-2 Protocol*).

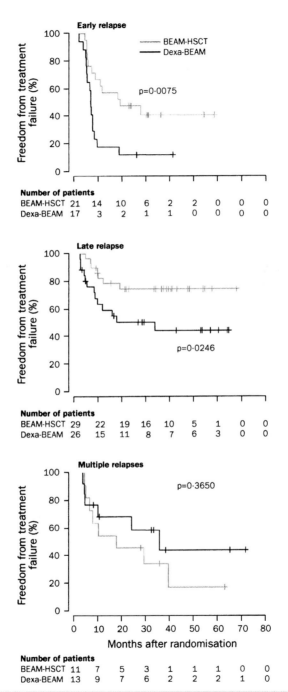

Fig. 2. FFTF for patients who have early relapse (*upper*), late relapse (*middle*), and multiple relapses (*lower*) of HL. HSCT, hematopoietic stem cell transplantation.

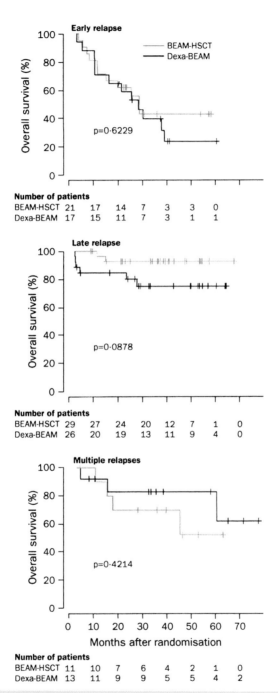

Fig. 3. Overall survival for patients who have early relapse (*upper*), late relapse (*middle*), and multiple relapses (*lower*) of HL. HSCT, hematopoietic stem cell transplantation.

Autologous Stem Cell Transplantation in Primary Refractory Disease

Prognosis of patients who have PRD, defined as progression during first-line chemotherapy or within 3 months of the end of therapy, is extremely poor. Nevertheless, and as opposed to non-Hodgkin's lymphoma, where chemorefractory patients are not salvaged by transplantation, even patients who fail first- and second-line chemotherapy may still enjoy a 20% to 30% chance of cure with ASCT.

The results of several single-institution studies and two large, retrospective, registry-based analyses suggest a superior outcome for patients who receive high-dose therapy and ASCT in this setting, but with noticeable differences from one study to another. In the EBMT analysis published by Sweetenham and colleagues [21], 175 PR-HL patients were presented; actuarial 5-year PFS and OS were 32% and 36%, respectively. In the Autologous Blood and Marrow Transplant Registry (ABMTR) analysis on 122 patients undergoing ASCT after an induction failure (IF) [22], actuarial probabilities at 3 years were 38% and 50% for PFS and OS, respectively. The reasons for these discrepancies are not clear, but one must be aware that under the definition of IF, different subsets of patients with different long-term outcomes can be included. In the ABMTR analysis, almost 50% of the patients whose response to salvage chemotherapy before ASCT was known had a chemosensitive disease before transplantation. Lazarus and colleagues [22] found that the presence of B symptoms at diagnosis and Karnofsky status at ASCT correlated with survival, and that the absence of these two factors was associated with an excellent 2-year survival of 87%. In the EBMT analysis [21], patients receiving more than one line of chemotherapy before transplantation did worse, in terms of OS and PFS.

The GEL/TAMO co-operative group presented the results of 62 patients treated with an ASCT for an IF [23]. One-year transplant-related mortality (TRM) was 14%. The response rate at 3 months after ASCT was 52% [CR in 21 patients (34%), PR in 11 patients (18%)]. Actuarial 5-year TTF and OS were 15% and 26%, respectively. The presence of B symptoms at ASCT was the only adverse prognostic factor significantly influencing TTF. The presence of B symptoms at diagnosis, MOPP-like regimens as first-line therapy, bulky disease at ASCT, and at least two lines of therapy before ASCT adversely influenced OS.

Fermé and colleagues [24], from the GELA, reported on 157 patients with either IF, PR of less than 75%, or relapse after doxorubicin-based chemotherapy ± radiotherapy. All patients received mitoguazone, ifosfamide, vinorelbine, and etoposide (MINE) as second-line therapy, followed by ASCT with BEAM as the preparative regimen. The 5-year OS rates were 30% for patients with IF versus 72% for patients with less than 75% PR, and 76% for patients with relapsed disease following first-line therapy. Of the 101 patients who went on to transplantation, the 5-year freedom from second failure rate for patients with a response to MINE was 64% versus 25% for those not responding to MINE. Of the 64 patients with IF, 40 responded to second- or third-line salvage therapy, and 32 of these patients went on to transplantation. Of the 24 patients not responding to salvage, 9 went on to transplantation, only 1 of whom achieved a CR with ASCT.

The long-term outcome of 75 consecutive patients who had biopsy-confirmed HL at the completion of primary chemotherapy or combined modality therapy has been summarized by the Memorial Sloan Kettering Cancer Center group [25]. All patients underwent standard-dose salvage therapy followed by involved field radiotherapy to sites of active disease. Patients without progression went on to receive high-dose etoposide, cyclophosphamide, and either total lymphoid irradiation (if no prior radiotherapy) or carmustine (if prior radiotherapy), followed by bone marrow or peripheral stem cell rescue. Seven patients were excluded from transplantation because of progression on standard salvage therapy and had a 4-month median survival. Patients with less than a 25% decrease with standard salvage therapy (n = 27) had a 10-year EFS of 17% versus 60% for those with at least a 25% decrease to standard second-line therapy (n = 48).

However, as indicated by all the previously shown analyses and as highlighted by Josting [26], reports of ASCT for PRD are subject to significant selection bias. Patients with rapidly progressive disease, poor performance status, older age, and poor stem cell harvest are not included in the reports. The GHSG, in a landmark analysis comparing patients with PRD who did or did not receive transplant within 6 months of progression, and excluding all patients who survived less than 6 months, showed no advantage to ASCT over those treated with conventional salvage therapy [26].

In conclusion, most large transplantation series continue to show that response to conventional chemotherapy pretransplantation is highly predictive of outcome. Patients who have PRD who respond to a second-line salvage regimen still have a reasonable outcome with ASCT. In this sense, the high-dose sequential protocol of the GHSG, which significantly increases the intensity of the salvage regimen before transplantation, demonstrates a FFTF and OS of 38% and 55%, respectively, in the group of patients treated for PRD [27]. Those with no response to first- or second-line therapy are candidates for new approaches such as an allogeneic stem cell transplantation (allo-SCT).

Preparative Regimen for Autologous Stem Cell Transplantation

No randomized trial has ever compared preparative regimens for transplantation for relapsed HL. The only recent article addressing this question was a retrospective review by investigators at the Fred Hutchinson Cancer Research Center. Between 1990 and 1998, 92 patients who had relapsed HL were transplanted with either a TBI-based regimen or busulfan/melphalan/thiotepa [28]. The choice of the preparative regimen was based primarily on whether or not the patient had a prior history of dose-limiting radiation. The study showed no difference in 5-year OS (57% versus 52%) or EFS (49% versus 42%) rates for patients treated with TBI or chemotherapy only. Older retrospective comparisons reported similar results. Given the reports of increased risk of second cancers and myelodysplasia following TBI, a chemotherapy-only preparative regimen is currently favored by most transplant centers [16].

Prognosis After a Failed Autologous Stem Cell Transplantation

The median survival for patients who have a relapse posttransplantation is approximately 2 years, with the most important predictor of outcome being response to salvage therapy [29,30]. The GEL/TAMO co-operative group recently reported the long-term outcome of a group of 175 patients who relapsed at a median time of 10 (4–125) months after ASCT [31]. At 3 years, OS and PFS were 35% ± 4% and 23% ± 4%, respectively. Advanced clinical stage at relapse and a short time interval between ASCT and relapse (≤12 months) were independent adverse prognostic factors for PFS. Patients with both features had 3-year PFS of 14%, compared with 48% for patients without either factor. Advanced clinical stage at relapse, extranodal disease, and hemoglobin level of less than or equal to 100 g/L at relapse were significant adverse prognostic factors for OS.

ALLOGENEIC STEM CELL TRANSPLANTATION IN REFRACTORY/RELAPSED HODGKIN'S LYMPHOMA

Myeloablative Conditioning and Allogeneic Stem Cell Transplantation in Hodgkin's Lymphoma

The first reports on allo-SCT in patients who had HL appeared in the mid-1980s [32,33]. Two larger registry-based studies published in 1996 gave disappointing results. Gajewski and colleagues [34] analyzed 100 HL patients allografted from HLA-identical siblings and reported to the International Bone Marrow Transplant Registry. The 3-year rates for OS and disease-free survival, and the probability of relapse, were 21%, 15%, and 65%, respectively. The major problems after transplantation were persistent or recurrent disease or respiratory complications, which accounted for 35% to 51% of deaths. Acute or chronic graft-versus-host disease (GVHD) did not significantly reduce the risk of relapse. A case-matched analysis including 45 allografts and 45 autografts reported to the EBMT was performed by Milpied and colleagues [35]. They did not find significant differences in actuarial probabilities of OS, PFS, and relapse rates between allo-SCT and ASCT (25%, 15%, 61% versus 37%, 24%, 61%, respectively). The actuarial TRM at 4 years was significantly higher for allografts than for autografts (48% versus 27%, $P = .04$). Acute GVHD greater than or equal to grade II was associated with a significantly lower risk of relapse, but also with a lower survival rate.

A number of reports confirmed the registry data: allo-SCT resulted in lower relapse rates but significantly higher toxicity, with no improvement over ASCT when PFS or OS were considered [36–38]. Although the poor results after myeloablative conditioning could be explained at least partly by the very poor-risk features of many individuals included in these early studies, the high procedure-related morbidity and mortality prevented the widespread use of allo-SCT.

Reduced-Intensity Conditioning and Allogeneic Stem Cell Transplantation in Hodgkin's Lymphoma

Since the first clinical experiences that suggested that allo-SCT after a reduced-intensity conditioning (RIC) (RIC/allo-SCT) might represent an interesting alternative to classic allo-SCT, a number of reports have addressed the question of whether RIC/allo-SCT might also work for patients who have HL. Although the overall number of patients with HL treated with allo-SCT has remained low in comparison to other hematologic malignancies, the percentage of patients with refractory and relapsed HL who received a RIC/allo-SCT has been growing steadily in Europe over the last 5 years (Fig. 4).

The largest cohort of patients treated with RIC/allo-SCT in HL was recently reported by the Lymphoma WP of the EBMT [39] and included 374 patients. Median time from diagnosis to allo-SCT was 41 (4–332) months. Patients had received an average of four lines of prior therapy (1–8), and 288 patients (77%) had failed one or two ASCT. At the time of allo-SCT, 79 patients (21%) were in CR, 146 patients (39%) had chemosensitive disease, and 149 (40%) had chemoresistant disease or untested relapse. Two hundred and thirty-four patients (63%) were allografted from a matched sibling donor (MRD), 112 (30%) from a matched unrelated donor (MUD), and 28 from a mismatched donor (7%). Grade II to IV acute GVHD was reported in 27% of patients, and chronic GVHD in 40% of patients at risk. The 100-day TRM was 12%, but it increased to 20% at 12 months, and to 22% at 3 years; it was significantly worse for patients who had chemoresistant disease. Two-year PFS was 29% and again was significantly worse for those with chemoresistant disease ($P<.001$). The development of chronic GVHD was associated with a higher TRM and a trend to a lower relapse rate. In a landmark analysis, the development of either acute or chronic GVHD by 9 months posttransplantation was associated with a significantly lower relapse rate.

The MD Anderson Cancer Center recently updated its experience [40] in 58 patients who had relapsed or refractory HL who underwent a

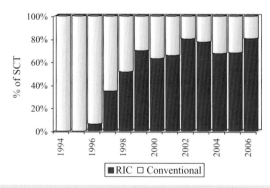

Fig. 4. Allo-SCT for relapsed and refractory HL. Comparison between conventional conditioning and RIC regimens. (*Courtesy of* the Lymphoma Working Party of the European Group for Blood and Marrow Transplantation, Maastricht, The Netherlands; with permission.)

RIC/allo-SCT from an MRD (n = 25) or a MUD (n = 33). Forty-eight (83%) patients had received a prior ASCT. Disease status at RIC/allo-SCT was sensitive relapse (n = 30) or refractory relapse (n = 28). The conditioning regimen used was fludarabine (125–130 mg/m^2 over 4–5 days) and melphalan (140 mg/m^2 IV over 2 days) (FM), and antithymocyte globulin (thymoglobulin 6 mg/kg over 3 days) was added for the 14 most recent MUD transplants. Cumulative 100-day and 2-year TRM were 7% and 15%, respectively. The cumulative incidence (CI) of grade II to IV acute GVHD was 28%. The CI of chronic GVHD at any time was 74%. Fourteen patients (24%) received a total of 25 (range 1–5) donor lymphocyte infusions (DLIs) for disease progression/relapse. Five of them (35%) also received chemotherapy, and nine (64%) developed acute GVHD after the DLI. Projected 2-year OS and PFS were 64% and 32%, respectively, with 2-year projected disease progression at 55%. MRD and MUD transplants showed no statistically significant difference with regard to OS, PFS, and disease progression. The response status before allo-SCT tended to impact PFS ($P = .07$) and disease progression ($P = .049$) favorably, but not OS ($P = .4$). Partial responders and patients who had stable/refractory disease fared similarly with regards to OS and PFS.

A study of 40 patients with relapsed or refractory HL treated with the combination of fludarabine (150 mg/m^2) and melphalan (140 mg/m^2) has recently been presented by the Spanish group [41]. GVHD prophylaxis consisted of cyclosporine A and methotrexate. Twenty-one patients (53%) had received more than two lines of chemotherapy, 23 patients (58%) had been irradiated, and 29 patients (73%) had failed a previous ASCT. Twenty patients were allografted in resistant relapse and 38 patients received hematopoietic cells from an MRD. One-year TRM was 25%. Acute GVHD developed in 18 patients (45%) and chronic GVHD in 17 (45%) of the 31 evaluable patients. Extensive chronic GVHD was associated with a trend to a lower relapse rate (71% versus 44% at 24 months, $P = .07$). The response rate 3 months after RIC/allo-SCT was 67%. Eleven patients received DLIs for relapse or persistent disease. Six patients (54%) responded. OS and PFS were 48% and 32% at 2 years, respectively. Refractoriness to chemotherapy was the only adverse prognostic factor for both OS and PFS.

Investigators from Seattle reported their results for 27 HL patients [42]. Eighteen patients had an MRD and nine had an MUD. The patients received 2 Gy TBI alone (n = 7) or in combination with fludarabine (90 mg/m^2), and immunosuppression consisted of micophenolate mofetil and cyclosporine A. All patients were heavily pretreated with a median of five prior regimens. Twenty-four patients had failed a previous ASCT. Before RIC/allo-SCT, 5 patients were in CR, 11 in PR, 4 had relapsed disease, and 7 had refractory disease. The overall incidence of grade II to IV acute GVHD was 52%. The incidence of extensive chronic GVHD was 55% at 1 year. Day 100 and 1 year TRM were 7% and 35%, respectively. One year OS, PFS, and relapse incidence were 51%, 18%, and 47%, respectively.

Peggs and colleagues [43] explored the effects of in vivo T-cell depletion with alemtuzumab followed by fludarabine (150 mg/m^2) and melphalan (140 mg/m^2) in multiply relapsed patients; 90% of them had failed a previous autograft. At transplantation, 8 patients were in CR, 25 patients were in PR, 1 patient was in untested relapse, and 15 had refractory disease. Thirty-one patients were allografted from an MRD and 18 from MUDs. All patients engrafted, grade II to IV acute GVHD occurred in 16% of patients, and 14% developed chronic GVHD before DLIs. Nineteen patients received DLIs for progression (n = 16) or mixed chimerism (n = 3). Nine patients (56%) showed a response, which was significantly associated with acute or extensive chronic GVHD. Nonrelapse mortality was 16% at 730 days. Projected 4-year OS and PFS were 56% and 39%, respectively. Clinical characteristics and outcomes of the mentioned studies are summarized in Table 1.

No definitive information is available with respect to the best conditioning protocol or the impact of T-cell depletion in this setting. If one accepts that attempting an effective graft-versus-HL reaction may require several months, preventing early progression by administering a vigorous conditioning regimen remains an essential goal still to be accomplished. In this sense, the combination of a more intensive preparative regimen, the BEAM protocol together with a profound T-cell depletion with alemtuzumab as acute GVHD prophylaxis, has been demonstrated to be associated with sustained donor engraftment, a high response rate, minimal toxicity (nonrelapse mortality 7.6%) and a low incidence of GVHD [44]. The two analyses presented by the Lymphoma WP of the EBMT also strengthen this argument. The use of TBI-based RIC protocols significantly increased disease progression after RIC/allo-SCT in Robinson's analysis [39], and TBI-based conditioning regimens also emerged as an adverse prognostic factor for disease progression after transplantation, PFS, and OS in the recently performed comparative analysis between conventional and RIC protocols [45].

Comparison of Myeloablative and Reduced-Intensity Conditioning Before Allogeneic Stem Cell Transplantation in Relapsed and Refractory Hodgkin's Lymphoma

The Lymphoma WP of the EBMT has performed the only analysis reported so far that compares outcomes after RIC or myeloablative conditioning and allo-SCT in patients with HL [45]. Ninety-seven patients with HL were allografted after RIC and 93 patients were allografted after a conventional regimen. A previous ASCT was more frequent in the RIC/allo-SCT group (59% versus 41%, $P = .03$), as was the use of peripheral blood stem cells (82% versus 56%; $P<.001$). Nonrelapse mortality was significantly decreased in the RIC/allo-SCT group [HR 2.43 (95% CI 1.48–3.98), $P<.001$]. PFS and OS were also better in the reduced-intensity group [HR 1.28 (95% CI 0.92–1.78), $P = .1$ and HR 1.62 (95% CI 1.15–2.28), $P = .005$]. The development of chronic GVHD significantly decreased the incidence of relapse after transplantation, which translated into a better PFS and OS. This analysis indicates that RIC/allo-SCT is able to